THE BODY CONNECTION

an Analog *Re-Boot* for Digital Times

Suzanna Hammond

First published by Ultimate World Publishing 2019
Copyright © 2019 Suzanna Hammond

ISBN

Paperback - 978-1-925884-46-3
Ebook - 978-1-925884-47-0

Suzanna Hammond has asserted her right under the Copyright, Designs and Patents Act 1988 to be identified as the author of this work. The information in this book is based on the author's experiences and opinions. The publisher specifically disclaims responsibility for any adverse consequences, which may result from use of the information contained herein. Permission to use information has been sought by the author. Any breaches will be rectified in further editions of the book.

All rights reserved. No part of this publication may be reproduced, stored in or introduced into a retrieval system, or transmitted in any form, or by any means (electronic, mechanical, photocopying, recording or otherwise) without the prior written permission of the author. Any person who does any unauthorised act in relation to this publication may be liable to criminal prosecution and civil claims for damages. Enquiries should be made through the publisher.

Cover design: Ultimate World Publishing
Layout and typesetting: Ultimate World Publishing
Editor: Marinda Wilkinson

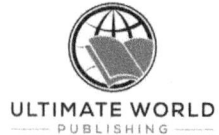

Ultimate World Publishing
Diamond Creek,
Victoria Australia 3089
www.writeabook.com.au

– What people are saying –

"I've known Suzanna Hammond since 1992. I value her practical, research-focused approach to investigation, diagnosis and treatment. As a client, I've found her truly masterful in the way she weaves her multiple healing modalities into a beautiful, specialised treatment for each person who is lucky enough to find her. This book will be a way for many more people to benefit from the down-to-earth wisdom she imparts during her treatments."

Dr E. Joy Bowles, PhD, BSc,
author, educator & researcher

"I love the gritty observations and common sense in this book! Like Suzanna, it's funny, informative and relevant to all ages. Challenges you to think about our throwaway quick fix society and how this new order is affecting our lives and health. Plus, her real life client stories are so encouraging."

Vivienne Neate,
publications assistant

"With her wealth of knowledge, experience, compassion and understanding a visit to Suzanna will focus, soothe and *unfrazzle* you. I'd come in crackling like an electrical storm and leave completely calm – all senses serenaded."

Jeni Mawter, author & educator

"I have managed to delay bilateral knee replacements for 17 years by following Suzanna's treatment plans of remedial strengthening and stretching exercises, attention to posture, dietary and lifestyle changes. Her practical assessments and extensive knowledge have ensured I always leave a session feeling very much better than when I came in."

Annette Livesey, company secretary

"Suzanna truly cares about each of her clients, their health and circumstances. A total mind, body, spirit therapist."

Diane Jenkins, IT specialist

"I first saw Suzanna as an aromatherapist after a traumatic car accident. I soon discovered she was also an amazing remedial bodywork therapist with a deep understanding of the human body and how it works. Years later I still use the techniques she taught me. With Suzanna's help, I feel I've avoided a future that would have seen me limited by my injuries."

Lotus Cavagnino, aged care worker

"I presented myself to Suzanna looking like a train wreck! Her holistic approach to fitness and wellbeing helped me regain my strength, confidence and avoid spinal surgery. I am forever grateful for her time and knowledge, which she openly shares."

Bronwyn Ugonotti, office administrator

"A friend recommended Suzanna a few years ago when I was suffering chronic back pain. Since then, Suzanna's aromatic remedial massage and hot stone therapy has headed off medical and surgical intervention for my knees and back."

Ann Buckley, registered nurse

"Suzanna was recommended to me as an excellent holistic aromatherapist who could help me with embarrassing skin problems I'd had since I was a teenager in the 70s. Unlike all the doctors and specialists I'd seen in the past, she closely examined my diet and environmental background. She discovered I'd grown up in the vicinity of a very toxic factory, for example. And that as the child of migrant parents I'd spent years trying to fit in with 'Anglo culture' by eating too much 'junk' food. Three months after tackling my skin problems with diet, skincare, aromatherapy facials and supplements, my friends at work were asking me what I was doing to make my skin look so good!"

Maria Laver, art teacher

"I've been treating myself to Suzanna's aromatic massages and rejuvenating facials for many years now and can highly recommend the experience. I believe her thoroughly pleasurable treatments and knowledgeable attention have kept my skin in great condition from my 70s through to my 80s."

Norma Cottrell, retired school administrator

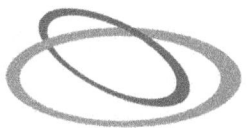

For Zosha & Bastiaan

"THERE IS MORE TO LIFE THAN SIMPLY INCREASING ITS SPEED."

Mahatma Gandhi

Contents

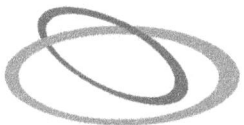

What people are saying iii
Dedication vii
Introduction xi
Chapter 1: Life on the Cutting Edge 1
Chapter 2: Exploding the 'Magic Silver Bullet' 7
Chapter 3: The 12 Vital Operating Systems
of the Analog Body 19
Chapter 4: The Power of REAL food 43
Chapter 5: When the Food Leaves the Fork:
My '3 Golden Rules' & Other Stories 55
Chapter 6: Bite on This 69
Chapter 7: You Gotta Have Skin 75
Chapter 8: Float Like a Butterfly: Surprising Links
Between Posture, Balance & Strength 91
Chapter 9: Move It … or Lose It! 103
Chapter 10: The Miracle of Touch 119
Chapter 11: RELAX! Nothing is Under Control 135
Chapter 12: And So, To Sleep… 143
Wellbeing is a journey, not an app 157
Further reading 158
About the Author 161
Acknowledgements 163

Introduction

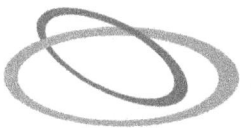

If you're reading this book, chances are you're already thinking that a few things in your life need to change.

Perhaps you've experienced poor health caused by unhealthy habits – especially overwhelm caused by too much self-inflicted busyness. Maybe you've been looking around you at the phones everyone carries everywhere, wondering when exactly did that become a thing? Or your smart house regularly comes to a grinding halt when lightning strikes or power cuts. Maybe you've started to wonder why people bother going out to restaurants together if they're going to spend the time scrolling through information on their phones that they won't even recall? Posting pictures of food they don't eat? Children glued to screens to shut them up instead of teaching them how to behave at the dinner table. How we've come to live our lives by the standards of brand-marketing and lifestyle hype, rather than using our innate common sense. And how we're all increasingly paying for our connectedness addiction with rising, entirely preventable physical and mental illness, toxic environments and the most wasteful societies our world has ever seen.

If you've found yourself wondering how we all got so disconnected in such a connected world… take heart, it's not too late to change. 'THE BODY CONNECTION' is a timely overview of how and why we've arrived at some of the alarming but preventable health statistics we're seeing today. And I'm here to inspire you to get back to some good old-fashioned *analog*-style basics. Read on.

Analog
(also spelled analogue)

Relating to or using signals or information
represented by a continuously variable physical quantity –
a continuous wave that keeps changing over a period of time.

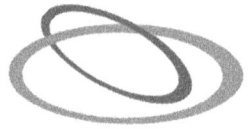

Digital

Signal or data expressed as series of the digits 0 and 1,
typically represented by values of a physical quantity
such as voltage or magnetic polarisation.
Using or storing data in the form of digital signals –
involving or relating to the use of computer technology.

CHAPTER 1

Life on the Cutting Edge

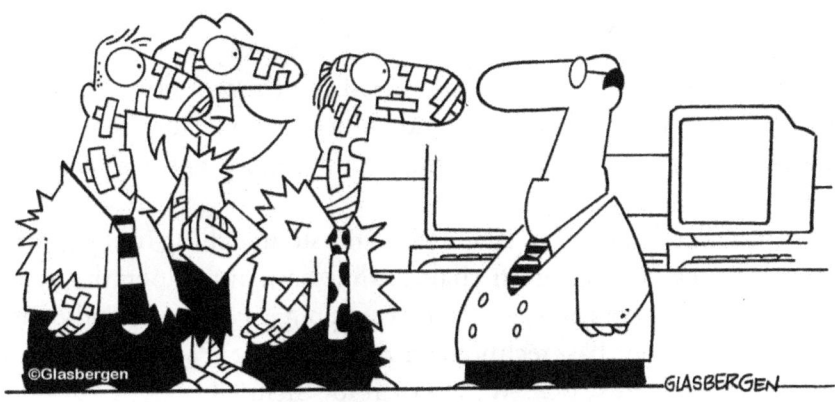

"Frankly sir, we're tired of being on the cutting edge of technology."

You've got to hand it to the trend forecasters. The built-in obsolescence of mortality may have claimed individuals but, just like the tsunami of wall-to-wall plastics they predicted in the 1960s, their madcap hypothetical gig has proved scarily durable. With a business model characterised by wishful thinking, flashy guesswork and zero responsibility, these opportunistic, corporate soothsayers *still* manage to straddle big business and social engineering with their peculiar and shameless oeuvre of marketing cunningly disguised as trend clairvoyance. In short, trend forecasters neither create nor produce, but they get paid squillions of bucks for telling us what we need before we know we need it. Nice work if you can get it.

Sophisticated as we think we are, you'd think we'd have seen through the siren-song of driftnet marketing by now, but no. As forecasting becomes more sophisticated, competitive, targeted and urgent, we're still falling over ourselves to be *first* (or at least, *early*) adopters of the next big thing. Reputations depend upon it. Keeping up with keeping up is vital. Never mind that we're drowning in stuff and our collective health is suffering. We must have it all because we can.

What if we all take a moment and look at a quick history of trend forecasting to get an idea of what a force this industry has become. And let's do it before we lose our health, minds, fine motor skills, intuitive instincts, native common sense and ability to think for ourselves to automation and the great profit churn of Big Corp Futures Inc.

Ever since trend-spotting surfaced as a measurable thing in the 1960s, the star-struck and movers 'n' shakers alike have hung upon the trend forecasting industry's every word. Fast shopping? Fast housework? Fast food? Fast fashion? Fast technology? Fast turnover? Fast growth? Fast medicine? Tick, tick, tick. We've fallen for them all.

You may not realise it, but all that was already happening way back in the day when many of you, dear readers, were not yet so much as a futuristic entry on your parents' to-do list. Those 'ancient history' days when white goods, packaged foods, cleaning products, additives, colourants, preservatives, fillers, plastic extrusions of every shape and size – including a raft of synthetic fabrics also derived from petrochemicals – became so profitable and highly desirable. And then slowly but surely insinuated themselves into our lives until, before we knew it, we couldn't do without them. All much to the delight of the shareholders of companies manufacturing millions of units of this and that for the brave new up-to-the-minute modern world.

Needless to say, the corporate soothsayers weren't telling us that they were just trying to get the economy going after World War 2 by selling us stuff we'd lived perfectly well without up until then. Or that, in order to secure jobs for returned WW2 soldiers and breed the next generation, the women who had been 'manning' the factories for the war effort needed to get back in the kitchen and stay there – as consumers of (and slaves to) the never ending roll-out of labour-saving devices and not-so-subtle feminine conduct protocols. Neither did anyone think to forecast that the 50s and 60s trend forecasts of ever-increasing profits might become locked into the corporate governance models we still operate under today and how we might find ourselves drowning in stuff just to keep it all going. Never mind what it might be doing to our health and communities. The marketing frenzy simply became the new way of doing business and we became sold on it.

To be entirely fair though, perhaps post-war enthusiasm for opportunity simply blinded everyone to either environmental consequences or social implications of this fabulously profitable way of thinking. How seductive, after years of hardship, was the glory of convenience? The glamour of gadgetry? Great expectations of new freedoms? The promise of status and upward mobility? How tempting the projection of an automatic, controllable and leisurely future – wherein we'd only work two or three days a week and leisure itself would emerge as the hot new business trend. Well, that's marketing for you!

Fifty or 60 years later – just as we were conned into believing the leisure and convenience promises of last century's trend gazers – we're becoming increasingly bamboozled and suckered in by the predictions delivered by the 21st century's hype spinners.

> *'Amazon CEO Jeff Bezos says there's a very simple reason his space company, Blue Origin, is working on a giant lunar lander to make moon travel as easy as an aeroplane flight: humanity's very survival relies on colonising space, starting with the moon... "The reason we've got to go into space, in my view, is to save the Earth," Bezos said. "We need to move heavy industry off the Earth. It will be way better done in space anyway. And Earth will be rezoned residential and light industry."'*
>
> **Julie Bort,**
> **'Make earth residential:**
> **Bezos wants to move factories to the moon',**
> *Sydney Morning Herald,* **7 June 2019**

Seriously? If this isn't a perfect example of Mad Tech, I'm damned if I know what is! Not content with becoming the richest man on earth by convincing us to buy stuff we don't need and then throw it away when we're tired of it, Bezos has chosen to apply his considerable genius to promoting yet another method of out of sight, out of mind outsourcing... this time to the moon! Never mind that the rest of us are struggling to manage the health of our own planet and our bodies are suffering from totally preventable diseases caused by our incessant and insatiable consumption of stuff. You'd have to be nuts to even imagine that a sensible solution would be to simply export our problems to other planets, right? Or seriously disconnected. Or maybe both.

Curiously, the one subject I've never heard any of the latest wave of marketing soothsayers discuss in public is the enormous *price* we are all paying for the latest incarnation of digital gadgetry, convenience, outsourcing and automation! Despite the fact that, as surely as night follows day, there is a hidden price for *everything*!

> *'You can have anything you want, as long as you accept that there is a price and that you will have to pay it.'*
> **Tana French,** ***The Likeness***

Take the ancient concept of landfill, for example. Once upon a time, people just dumped their refuse in a heap somewhere close to the village and called it a *midden*. With plastics, batteries and smart devices yet to be invented, only tools, bones and metal objects would be found five or ten or forty thousand years on. Because both people and food were scarce, little was wasted and there were scant greenhouse gases emanating from the pile. But fast-forward to any time after 1955 and we began to have a growing problem with where to dump our obsolete gadgets, machinery, cars and plastics and we slowly adopted an out of sight, out of mind attitude to where it was all going. That is, we stuck it somewhere we couldn't see it – and because our wasteful extravagance wasn't staring us in the face every day, *ipso facto*, it didn't exist. The important thing was to keep the wheels of industry turning by acquiring the next shiny thing. Consequently, nobody gave too much thought to where all our garbage was going until (60 or so years later) the Chinese announced that they weren't going to take any more of Australia's garbage in 2017! Then the Malaysians announced they weren't taking any more of our garbage in 2019. What the…? Who even knew before those under-reported moments that the Chinese and Malaysians were dealing with our garbage for us, anyway? Who was even vaguely interested in the logistics of where our convenience-addicted, plastic throwaway society was chucking their ever-increasing piles of rubbish and cast-off labour-saving machinery? The spent plastics, chemicals, clothing, poisons, computers, mobile phones, batteries, washing machines, clothes dryers, microwaves, fridges and wasted food all bubbling and disintegrating away, out of sight in distant (and sometimes illegal) landfill dumps across the country and, latterly, the world. In fact, how many people do you know personally who even think of where all our garbage goes even now?

So, what has any of this got to do with the *analog* rebooting of your health in digital times, I hear you ask? Plenty, actually.

All the above represents only a tiny summary of how we've arrived at where we are today in regard to ourselves as consumers, our immediate environments and our planet. And, as I sit typing this chapter on my desktop computer, I am utterly grateful that I'm not doing my cuts and pastes like Jane Austen in the 18th century – on parchment with bits of fabric and paper and pins. So, I'm definitely not saying that all progress and all vision is bad because it patently isn't. What I am saying is that we need to start thinking things through when it comes to what we're encouraged to believe is progress. Now, more than ever, we need to understand that we have a collective responsibility for the choices we make. And that includes the increasingly dire social, environmental and health costs of our indulgent but surprisingly stressful lifestyles.

In regard to our health – which is, after all, what this book is about – the good news is Australians are living longer than ever before because of foresight and innovation. The bad news? Most of us are taking our good fortune for granted and throwing away the best in favour of the next shiny thing. Sadly, we're so busy and attached to our screens that fewer than one person in a hundred has the faintest notion of how their body works or the simple things it really needs.

So, let's all take a light-hearted review of where we all are, health-wise, right now. You don't have to be or look perfect. Your age doesn't matter. Neither does your gender. What matters is that the sooner you begin to make some commonsense *analog* changes to connect with your own body and its needs, the better you'll feel.

This book is about the enduring magic of old-fashioned know-how. A top-to-toe holistic guide and kick up the backside to inspire you to take better care of yourself. The information you're about to read does not pretend to be the be-all and end-all of self-care – although for many it will be eye-opening and a damned fine start. We may live in strange times but achievable everyday miracles are right under our noses.

My own canny trend forecast is that you will be among the first to jump aboard the latest trend to profoundly connect with the miracle that is your body. And, while you're at it, come to understand the importance of extending that care to your living, breathing planet.

I look forward to sharing this *analog* journey with you.

CHAPTER 2

Exploding the 'Magic Silver Bullet'

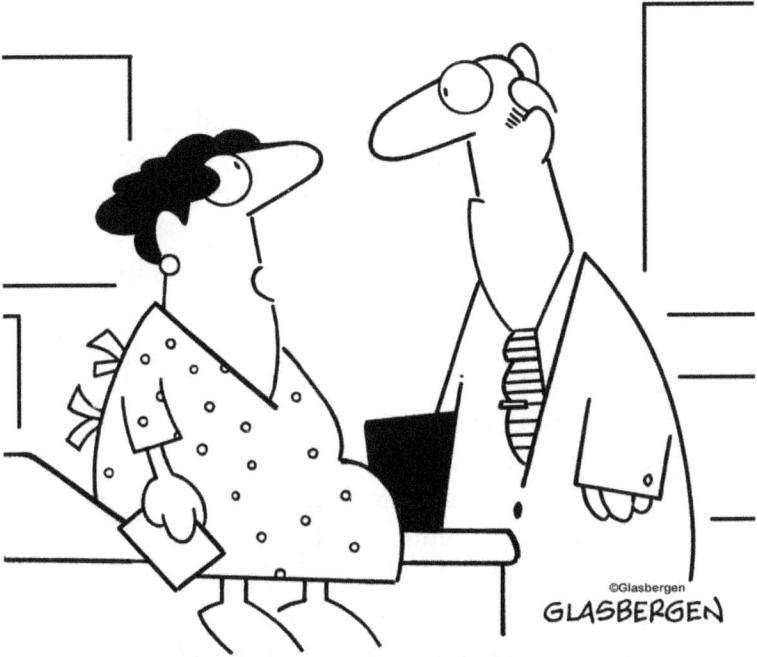

"I already diagnosed myself on the Internet. I either have three left kidneys, recurring puberty or Dutch Elm disease."

It's the middle of the night in the middle of nowhere. There's a full moon. An unnatural fog. And you. Up to your 'pussy's bow' in werewolves. Fresh out of 'if onlys', you resort to praying for the one mythical solution guaranteed to blast all your hairy problems into kingdom come. The single shiny thingamajig to which werewolves have had a majorly fatal vulnerability since Gilgamesh's day. Silver!

In its modern form as a MAGIC SILVER BULLET! 'Btw, Lord,' you cry out in the darkness of the moment, 'can you make that fast, instant and preferably retrospective? For I have places to go, people to see and shit to do!'

Years ago, pre-meme age, I wore a lapel badge which said, *'Sudden prayers make God jump!'*. Looking back, the message was prescient. Especially, when you consider how our expectations and addiction to effortless and fast solutions have speeded up in the wake of the internet, medical technology and the staggering array of magical thinking packaged and evangelised by the beauty and enlightenment industries. You're worth it, after all. But how, precisely, did we come to rely on a concept known as the 'magic silver bullet'?

Belief in the magical powers of silver is ancient. However, what is now referred to as the magic silver bullet has been upgraded, re-imagined and weaponised in line with available technology and even trade development throughout the ages. Once upon a time, it was just plain old magical, mystical silver that despatched werewolves, vampires, demons and other beings of the dark side. Then around 23BC *Horace's Odes* posited that no less than the Oracle of Delphi had advised Philip of Macedonia to fight with silver spears to gain advantage on the battlefield. The technological upgrade to silver bullets dates from the late 17th century. Around the same time that Christian Europeans were employing lead bullets to devastate entire populations of assumed godless, non-Christian indigenous populations as they pillaged, plundered and claimed the so-called 'New World' for themselves. These 17th century references broadened the efficacy of the silver bullet for use against the Devil himself, as well as his diverse gang, and continued through into popular 19th century fiction. It was only at the beginning of the 20th century that it began to expand and be adopted for use as a solution to problems in other contexts. For example – the 'Silver Bullet' war bonds of 1914 offered for investment with a fail-proof promise to safeguard and maximise savings. Although, I'm not sure what problem Harry Craddock was seeking to solve when he listed his 'Silver Bullet Cocktail' recipe in his 1930 *Savoy Cocktail*

Book. (Half gin, quarter lemon juice, quarter kummel. Shake well and strain into cocktail glass.)

The term 'magic bullet' was launched into medical usage in the early 20th century, coined by the German scientist and Nobel laureate Paul Ehrlich in 1906. While working at the Institute of Experimental Therapy, Ehrlich formed an idea that it could be possible to kill specific microbes that cause disease without harming the body itself. He named his hypothetical agent by the German word *zauberkugel* – or magic bullet. A report of Ehrlich's work in the August 1924 edition of *Science* stated:

> *'Ehrlich aptly compared them (natural antibodies) to magic bullets, constrained by a charm to fly straight to their specific objective, and to turn aside from anything else in their path.'*

His continued research to find and define his magic bullet resulted in the discovery of much new information about the workings of the body's immune system and the first effective drug for the scourge of syphilis (1909). His works were the foundation of the medical specialty known as immunology and for his contributions he shared the 1908 Nobel Prize in Physiology or Medicine with Elie Metchnikoff.

Medical use aside, at some point the idea of a miraculous butt-saving breakthrough became 'a magic silver bullet', the term now generally understood to refer to some widget, medication, concept or action which promises to cut through complexity and provide an immediate solution to a particularly difficult problem. And don't think the marketing people haven't noticed! These days we conceive, manufacture, tout and open our wallets wide in the hope of magic silver bullets for pretty much everything: business and banking, agriculture, urban design, product and policy development, politics and corporate governance, pharmaceuticals and herbal supplements – the list goes on!

In fact, nowadays we've got magic silver bullets of one sort or another 'up the yah-zoo', as one of my colleagues amusingly refers to overkill. We've become so accustomed to the idea that there will always be a magic silver bullet to vanquish whatever is giving us grief, we've come to think of the mere *concept* of it as a guarantee of its commonplace existence and free availability. In essence, we've come to believe in the sizzle rather than the steak.

Frankly, we're gagging on the magic silver bullets spawned by what we quaintly refer to as innovation, disruption and globalisation. There's a magical silver bullet (or at least two in development and seeking investors) for everything. Dicky heart or liver? Get a transplant. Wobbly knees or hips? Get some titanium joints. Sky high cholesterol? Take some statins. When it's finally broke – just fix it and move on. Maybe there's even an app. It'll cost you but it's effortless, don't you know? Like flicking a switch or changing a channel. Right? So how is it that – with all our civilisation and technology – we're fast losing even the remnants of our innate common sense and talent for bullshit detection? Why are we moving at warp speed towards losing our ability to discriminate between fact and fiction? Who convinced us it's perfectly normal to *outsource* everything because *we* surely don't have time? How did we get so busy being busy? And what price convenience if it's killing you?

Sure, you can blame the Biggies – Big Money, Big Development, Big Food, Big Sugar, Big Pharma, Big Techno, Big Booze, Big Petroleum, Big Plastic, Big Coal and their slew of stakeholders, advertising, PR and political flunkies – for the state of misinformation and corporate doublespeak all you like. You can mutter darkly about fake news and lazy media who publish entire corporate press releases holus-bolus for public consumption with neither editing nor fact checking in their efforts to feed their websites and ailing hard copy pages. You can shake your fists at multilevel marketing companies spruiking get-rich-quick hype through magical fixits (from cosmetics and cleaning agents to essential oils) for the under-employed to eke out a meagre profit as they upsell their friends. You can throw rocks at your TV. But nothing will make the teensiest bit of difference in the battle to *keep it real* until we stop believing the sales hype. And simply stop *buying* into it.

> *'What we're doing now is unsustainable. The only thing we can hope is that a sense of urgency will permeate. We're running out of time.'*
>
> **William Dietz,**
> **public health expert & an author of**
> **the 2019 EAT-Lancet Commission's report warning of**
> **the dangers of obesity, unsustainable agricultural**
> **production, transport, urban design and land use**

Isn't it time we made the choice to start checking the facts against what we so desperately want to believe will save us? And, in particular, that someone or *something* else is in charge of our own health and wellbeing? Because until then making conscious healthy choices for ourselves, our families and our planet… is just a pipedream.

> *'Malnutrition, be it under nutrition or obesity, is by far the biggest cause of ill-health and premature death globally.'*
>
> **Professor Steven Allender,**
> **EAT-Lancet obesity commissioner &**
> **director of the Global Obesity Centre at Deakin**
> **University's Institute for Health Transformation**

Of course, you can swipe left, hit the fatalism button and say none of it really matters in the end. We're all going to hell in a handbasket anyway, right? Why not indulge your sweet tooth, choose convenience over awareness, or whatever? But if you are still secretly banking on a magic silver bullet to save you when your own health and wellbeing go pear-shaped… how about we start with YOU! What if it's YOU that's the ultimate magic silver bullet?

What if YOU could upgrade and repair your long-suffering *analog* operating systems by reprogramming yourself with some astonishingly useful, reparative operational data? And I'm not only talking about reducing your carbon footprint and contribution to the mountains of plastic micro beads contaminating the food chain in your lifetime. I'm talking about what you can start doing today which will make you healthier overall – no matter what shape you're in. What if YOU could renovate YOU?

THE BODY CONNECTION

'It is worth pointing out that many patients who are afraid of becoming sick and possibly dying nevertheless do not take those measures which are known to lessen the risks of cancer and heart disease and many of the debilitating diseases of middle and old age... the exaggerated worry that characterises health anxiety is partly a response to a sense of helplessness in the face of danger.'

Dr Fredric Neumann,
***Psychology Today*, 28 December 2013**

One of the sticking points I've heard over the years runs like this – 'But how? I'm not a doctor. I don't even understand medical language.' And my response to it mostly goes something like this: 'Well, neither am I a doctor, as it happens. I'm a people renovator'. Albeit with 35 years of training and practice in many different modalities of bodywork. Plus, a bucket load of good old-fashioned common sense, courtesy of my Yorkshire grandmother.

Over the years I've had to acquire a working knowledge of all sorts of medical and pharmaceutical terms. As a writer of pharmaceutical advertising and information for the medical profession. As a creator/producer of perinatal and women's health films. To liaise with GPs, medical specialists, physiotherapists and mental health professionals in my job as a bodywork therapist. And to troubleshoot my own medical emergencies, for example, post-viral syndrome, breast cancer, a particularly nasty battle with a hiatal hernia and severe medication induced anaemia. It won't hurt you to know what medications you're taking, their side effects and why you're taking them in the first place. And it surely won't kill you to learn some medical language either. It's not that hard once you get the hang of it. Don't be intimidated by the Latin – even the Romans had trouble with it!

Understanding at least some of the medical terms relevant to your own health and how to ask your doctor to explain things to you in plain English are two of the first baby steps of becoming your own health advocate.

In any case, most of what you need to start doing today doesn't require medical language at all. So maybe just start small and:

- Stop wasting time, procrastinating and/or waiting for the miracle to come

- Get curious about your health and how you can improve it

- Read trustworthy sources about conditions you're suffering

- Start making basic lifestyle improvements one at a time

- Read the rest of this book to see how else you can start tuning into your body and contributing to your own health care plan.

'The consequences of rising obesity extend beyond the waistline. This means our risk of diabetes, heart attacks, stroke, reflux and many cancers including oesophageal, bowel, breast and liver cancers have all increased dramatically.'
**Dr Adrian Sartoretto,
gastroenterologist at The BMI Clinic**

The other question I hear a lot is, 'Isn't getting me in better health the job of my health care practitioner?' to which I usually quite heartlessly reply – 'Actually, your overall health is *your* job!'.

Because your health care professional's job starts when you walk in their door and tell them what's going on with you. As *you* see it. No matter how overwhelmed or uneducated you think you are. Then, hopefully, they start working with you (and you start working with them) to either fix or manage whatever is less than ideal. If you're not getting that kind of service, you should be looking for another health care professional. But if you're not bringing your commitment with you, there's not that much they can do for you. If you're slowly undermining your own health and wellbeing with your lifestyle choices the road back to health may be a very long one.

In essence, that's what this entire book is about. Because we may all be living longer but the statistics tell us we're now plagued by *preventable* diseases. For example:

- 1 in 2 Australians will be diagnosed with cancer by the age of 85[1]

- 1 in 2 Australians over the age of 16 will experience mental illness[2]

- 2 in 3 adults and more than a quarter of children are overweight or obese[3]

- 1 in 5 people aged 25 to 54 say they don't have time to look after their health[4].

In any case, with almost 50% of chronic illness now entirely preventable, doesn't it make sense to clean up your act before the proverbial brown stuff hits the proverbial blades and it's too little too late even if there is a magic silver bullet?

Before we finish this chapter, let's take a look at a real-life example of what can happen when you show up as your own *magic silver bullet*...

---

[1] Australian Institute of Health and Welfare 2019, 'Cancer in Australia: In brief 2019' *Cancer Series*, no.122.

[2] Australian Institute of Health and Welfare 2018, 'Australia's Health 2018', *Australia's Health Series*, no.16.

[3] Summary Report of the EAT-*Lancet* Commission 2019.

[4] Strazdins, L & Venn D 2016, 'Household, Income and Labour Dynamics in Australia (HILDA) Survey'.

EXPLODING THE 'MAGIC SILVER BULLET'

A few years ago, one of my 'injury rehab' clients referred a badly injured young friend to me, hoping I could get him out of the doldrums. A couple of years prior, she had employed me to help her rehabilitate a badly broken ankle, following a fall off a slippery log into a ravine. Months of immobilisation in a 'moon boot' had sapped the bushwalker's strength in her legs, given her all kinds of pain from muscular compensations as she hobbled about and all confidence in her balance was shot. She knew I was bossy about form and practice, could execute a soothing massage when pain was unbearable and had a pretty offbeat sense of humour to boot. Best of all, she knew my methods worked – after finally committing to do her strength and balance routines *daily*, she'd recovered said strength and balance and was planning to walk the Camino de Santiago.

The young man, I'll call him Paul, had been left with a smashed and mangled right lower leg and ankle when a boulder fell on him in a climbing accident. His muscle and skin injuries were horrendous. Because the accident had occurred in a remote location it was touch and go whether he would bleed out before a rescue helicopter could fly him to a hospital. But his luck was in. He was transfused in the nick of time. He'd managed to reach a hospital with a brilliant orthopaedic surgical team. The skin graft team and facilities were outstanding. The various surgical teams took a bit of bone from his pelvis, and sliced muscle and skin from his back, buttocks and thighs. Over more than a dozen surgeries those brilliant teams used the tissues to gradually patch and repair the damage and avoid having to amputate his injured leg.

Paul turned up at my studio a year later, dropped off by a mate. The young man I saw was very much alive, but he thought his life was over. He was 25 and looked like he'd come off badly in a stoush with a white pointer. The surgeons had done a marvellous job, but his leg still look liked a patchwork of tissue. His ankle was off at a peculiar angle. Fortunately, the tissue harvesting sites on his back and legs had healed and the scars were fading. But weight bearing, even on crutches, was excruciating. He couldn't walk or drive, so he couldn't work. He was also battling constant recurrent staph infections in the bone graft sites and glugging down the most potent antibiotics available daily, month after month.

THE BODY CONNECTION

Paul had assumed that 12 months after his accident, he'd be back to normal. Instead, he was exhausted, downhearted and constantly nauseous from the antibiotics. On his first visit, he told me with some certainty that he would never be able to attract a girlfriend again. 'I hate this bloody leg,' he said with raw anger and grief. 'Sometimes, I wish they'd just taken the bloody thing off!'

And that was where we started. The situation was both fluid and complex. Nevertheless, a treatment plan gradually unfolded over the next few months.

The first priority was to relieve some of the pain in Paul's body to relax and help him regain some of the mental resilience which had made him an intrepid climber. He wasn't optimistic 'a bit of aromatherapy' would help him but he was out of options. We began with a combination of gentle neuromuscular massage applied with analgesic/anti-inflammatory essential oils like German chamomile and the legendary wound healers and protectors, frankincense and myrrh. During this process I also discovered that, aside from surgeons and nurses, no-one, not even *he*, had touched his wounds. In fact, he tried pretty hard not to even think about them, he said, especially that 'damned leg'.

This information led to the second part of the healing strategy – to reconnect Paul's mind to his injured leg. All somatic body workers know that withdrawing attention from an injury impedes the healing process. We also know that applying attention in a meditative process can increase blood flow to the injured area. So, I taught him to imagine balls of whatever coloured light he fancied, rolling along his leg for 10 minutes twice a day. More often, if he felt like it. A few sessions later he noticed his pain was lessening.

The next discipline to be applied was a gentle introduction to weight bearing straight out of Grandmaster Gary Khor's Tai Chi Falls Prevention Training exercises. We began with the simple but deceptively complex exercise of shifting body weight from side to side through the legs, engaging Paul's complete attention to how his body was reacting. A few sessions later Paul was able to start lifting his injured leg while he stood on the other. Then, very slowly, he began to shift his weight to his injured leg while holding on to a bench. Within a couple of months, he was able to extend his strength and balance training to riding a bike. Then he found a job that he could get to on his bike. The more he cycled the stronger and happier he became. He cleaned up his diet. He took probiotics in between antibiotic doses. He made sure his diet was full of *pre*biotics too – the types of fibre your good gut bacteria thrive on.

It was time to work towards a bigger goal. One day he asked me if I thought he'd ever be able to run again because he'd been a keen participant in a city fun run for years until his accident. 'You might not be able to run the 14km. And you definitely won't finish in a world-stopping time,' I told him, 'but you could power walk it if you train properly. Oh, and you'll need to take someone with you to put you in a wheelchair, if it all goes south.'

And so, training began in earnest with more cycling. Posture strengthening exercises to reduce compensations and undue weight on his injured leg. More coloured balls of light. And more Tai Chi falls prevention exercises, this time in the form of the exquisitely slow discipline of Tai Chi walking on all kinds of surfaces and inclines.

Six months later, on a glorious pre-spring Sunday, Paul walked Sydney's City to Surf with a mate pushing his crutches, a supply of snacks and water in a wheelchair. He didn't come first. He didn't come last. He just showed up as his own *magic silver bullet*.

And some years later, he showed up on my doorstep unexpectedly to show me pictures of his wedding and introduce me to his beautiful little daughter.

CHAPTER 3

The 12 Vital Operating Systems of the Analog Body

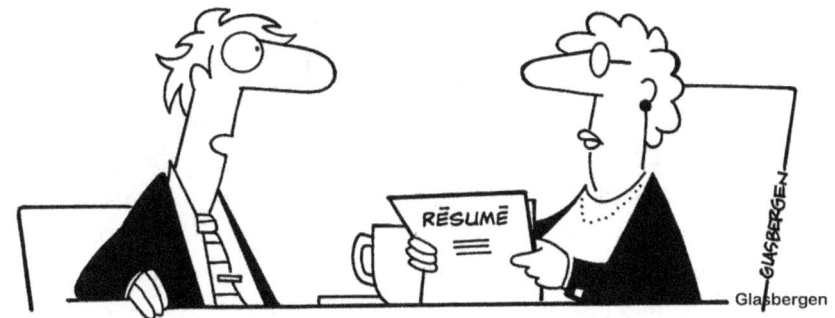

"I'm an expert at multitasking. I can digest food, grow hair, circulate blood, repair cells, make saliva, breathe, blink, walk and talk, all at the same time!"

Why is it that most of us have a *zip zero* level of either knowledge or interest in how our bodies work? And how is it that our cluelessness about our own anatomy and physiology persists despite the fact that we are practically drowning in wellness information pumped out daily on the portable smart-screens in front of us?

Think about it for a few moments. How much do you really know about what's going on beneath that marvellously practical, hold-all 'skin bag' that you've come to think of as YOU? And why should you even care about the bits you can't see? Surely, it's not *your* job?

Given most people take their bodies for granted until something goes wrong, maybe for the sake of your general health and wellbeing it's about time it was your job. And if you're thinking of flipping or scrolling or swiping past this chapter at this point, allow me to clarify. Maintaining a wilful ignorance about your own body can aggravate symptoms and lead to serious health problems in the future. Deliberate ignorance of basics can even suck you down the internet's bottomless rabbit hole of DIY 'cures', potions and fads and end up making the situation worse. I'm not suggesting you take a degree in functional anatomy. I'm simply talking about getting a functional overview of yourself. A working knowledge of how you work.

Often, when I start working with a new client to renovate some aspect of themselves, I'm flabbergasted by two things. Firstly, how very little they know about the basics of how their bodies work. Secondly, how many weird and wonderful so-called 'wellness tips' they can spout by heart from scrolling through the shedload of dodgy sites on the internet. It staggers me that, in the 'information age', we are still susceptible to the idea of investing our time and money in online 'snake oil' marketing schemes with catchy headlines and golden promises. Effectively outsourcing our learning and knowledge about our own bodies and health problems to advertising copywriters who are trained to sell us hope, quick fixes and, ultimately, stuff. (I know quite a lot about advertising copywriters because, back in the day, I used to *be* one!)

When it comes to our bodies, most of us think we know how to take care of ourselves. However, in reality, we rarely do so. It may come as something of a shock to learn that doctors, nurses and other health professionals are frequently just as bad as the rest of us in this regard. Knee-jerking their way through pain and discomfort. Ignoring red flags. Putting off regular health checks. Flicking through mindless stuff on the internet late at night in an attempt to relax their over-stimulated brains. You know the drill.

If you've been experiencing niggling symptoms such as headaches, constipation, joint pain and fatigue – especially, alarming and unusual discomforts that you've been trying to ignore – it's time to start listening to your body because it's trying to tell you something.

THE 12 VITAL OPERATING SYSTEMS OF THE ANALOG BODY

In fact, tuning into your body's messages may just save your life – just as tuning into my own body has saved my life on a number of occasions.

Over the next few pages you'll find an 'anatomical systems starter kit' to help you start paying attention to whichever part of your body is trying its darnedest to communicate with you. I'm not reproducing *Gray's Anatomy*. Or even a potted version of it. Just a brief, simplified, practical and accessible overview of the vital systems that keep the miracle of YOU going day after day, over a lifetime. So, find a comfortable spot, switch your phone to silent and settle in for an intriguing voyage through the operating systems of your own inner world.

Put simply, your body's systems are groups of organs, glands and tissues that perform important jobs and ideally work together to keep you going. Some organs and tissues may even be part of more than one body system if they serve more than one function. Helpfully, some of your body's systems even replace themselves every seven to 15 years! And if that snippet of information doesn't put a spring in your step, maybe the following confirmation of what a miracle of a body you're travelling in will.

The **SKELETAL** System

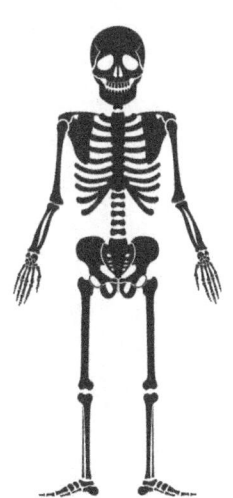

Your skeleton is the internal framework of your body. At birth we start off with 270 bones, some of which fuse together as we grow into adulthood when our bone count decreases to 206 bones. You may be surprised to know that your skeleton completely regenerates itself approximately every 10 years!

Your bones are connected together by strappy ligaments and a firm but flexible protective connective tissue at the joints called cartilage. Cartilage can bend a bit but resists stretching. Cartilage is also found in the rib cage, ears, nose, throat and between the vertebrae of your spine.

The bones of your skeleton serve many important functions – from protecting your internal organs to giving your body support, allowing you the leverage to move and generally carrying you around. And, as if your bones don't work hard enough for you already, deep inside them, the spongy tissue of your bone marrow is busy making the stem cells that will generate new red blood cells to help your circulatory system carry oxygen through your body, white blood cells to help your immune system fight infection and platelets that help with blood clotting. Whew!

Because these days we expect to live well into our 80s and beyond, it can be a bit disappointing to learn that our bone mass reaches maximum density at around 21 years of age. But take heart! Before you start thinking that your best days are already (or close to being) behind you, go to Chapter 9 and read how movement and weight bearing exercise can increase bone density at any age.

You can help keep your skeletal system healthy by performing weight bearing exercise, weight training, eating calcium and magnesium rich foods in addition to a nutritious diet, adding vitamin D to your day in the form of sunshine and supplementation (if necessary), avoiding excessive alcohol, balance training to avoid falls and having your bone density tested at 50 or before.

The MUSCULAR System

Mostly, your body's muscles operate to move you, stimulate movement in your internal organs and keep your heart going. They fall into three main categories – skeletal, visceral and cardiac. But the 'busiest' muscles in the human body are actually the extraocular muscles, the eye muscles. The extraocular muscles are small, strong and efficient. Humans have six of them in each eye and these six muscles are constantly moving the eye about in order to follow whatever it is we're looking at. (No wonder our eyes get tired with all that swiping and scrolling!)

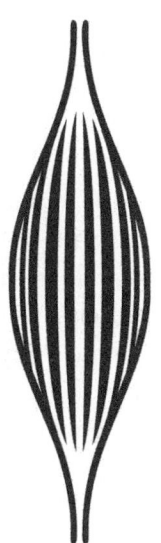

Skeletal muscle (or striated muscle) supports, protects and enables your skeleton to walk, run, jump, dance, cycle, pole vault, balance, lift heavy stuff and everything else you do that requires movement and functional strength. Skeletal muscles help stabilise your joints, maintain your posture and generate heat during activity. They also help maintain your body's temperature, burn fat, facilitate your circulation and, with movement, help your lymphatic system to drain interstitial fluids from the tissues.

Skeletal muscles are attached to your bones by tendons and work by contracting or extending. For example – when you lift a dumbbell your biceps contract and your triceps extend; when you slowly put it down again, your biceps extend and your triceps contract. Unless you drop it, of course – in which case nothing much is working! Which brings me to the next point that skeletal muscle is (or should be) completely under the control of the conscious nervous system, or *somatic* nervous system.

Smooth muscle (involuntary or visceral muscle), on the other hand, is generally under the control of your subconscious, or *autonomic* nervous system, the workings of which we are mostly blissfully unaware. In a few cases, smooth muscle can be controlled by the conscious mind. Yogis, some meditators and martial artists sometimes learn how to do this, but it takes disciplined practice, awareness and training. Nevertheless, for most people, the functions of smooth muscle are mostly completely automatic.

Smooth muscle covers many of your internal organs and is found in the walls of hollow organs such as your stomach, oesophagus, bronchi, as well as in the walls of your blood and lymphatic vessels. Smooth muscle is intricately involved in many of the housekeeping functions of your body. For example – it's responsible for holding certain passage shut. Like your anus, urethra and your lower oesophageal sphincter which works in tandem with your gastro oesophageal flap valve to prevent acid reflux. (So many folks are plagued with acid reflux! Bolted food, hours hunched over your screen and high stress levels don't help matters either.)

Smooth muscle in the uterus helps a woman to push out her baby during the birth process. In the bladder, smooth muscle helps push out urine. Its elasticity determines the flow and pressure of blood in your arteries. It is responsible for erecting the hair on your arms, head and the back of your neck, and the 'goosebumps' response.

Cardiac muscle is found only in your heart. Cardiac muscle could be described as a cross between smooth and striated muscle, insofar as it resembles skeletal muscle in form but, like smooth muscle, its function is involuntary.

Cardiac muscle cells are specialised to pump blood efficiently and continually throughout your entire lifetime. Ideally, without stopping for a rest, even when *you* need one. Given its workload – cardiac muscle is second only in its energy and nutrient requirements to your brain – it's just as well that your cardiac muscle has a miraculous ability to resist fatigue. Astonishingly, cardiac muscle cells have far more *mitochondria* per cell than hardworking skeletal muscle or any other type of cell or organ in your body! Often referred to as the powerhouses of the cell, mitochondria are the parts of all cells that turn sugars, fats and proteins into forms of chemical energy that your body can use to carry on living. Be grateful that your heart has such a phenomenal number of these tiny powerhouses and is so determined to keep you alive. But never take it for granted.

You can help keep your muscular system healthy by exercising regularly, warming up and cooling down before and after exercise, mindful stretching, eating a nutritious diet, keeping yourself hydrated, and with proper rest and recovery.

The INTEGUMENTARY and EXOCRINE System

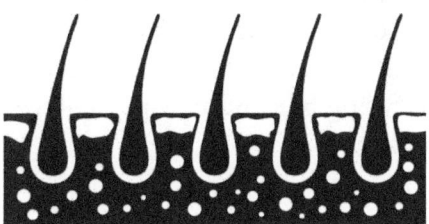

Bad hair day? Flaky nails? Shiny face? Oily skin? Sweating like a trooper? Blame it on what's going on with your integumentary and exocrine systems! As a fellow anatomy student once remarked, 'Blimey, Suze, it seems like all we do is ooze and seep…'. She might have added that between them, these two systems also cause much of the angst surrounding superficial grooming and beauty dilemmas.

Basically, the integumentary system consists of your skin, hair and nails – with the addition of your skin's sweat and sebaceous exocrine glands.

The two main components of the Integumentary system are the skin (epidermis, dermis and hypodermis) and its appendages (hair, nails, sweat and sebaceous glands), as well as associated muscle and nerve tissue. Although your skin is only a few millimetres thick, is it by far the largest organ of your body, accounting for between 12 to 15% of your total body weight. The skin's basic function is to protect your body from various kinds of damage such as loss of water and other kinds of external attack, like pathogens and injury. It contains sensory receptors, assists in the production of vitamin D, and plays a role in excretion and absorption. (See Chapter 7 for more information on your skin and how to look after it.)

Exocrine system is a system of glands that produce and secrete an astonishing array of protective and otherwise helpful substances onto your epithelial surfaces via tiny channels called ducts. Epithelial tissues line the outer surfaces of organs and blood vessels throughout your body – as well as the inner surfaces of the cavities in many internal organs. The most obvious and easy to see example of epithelium is the epidermis – the outermost layer of your skin – for which your sweat and sebaceous glands produce sweat and oil (sebum).

Other examples of the external exocrine system include – lacrimal (tears), ceruminous (earwax) and mammary glands (breast milk). While inside there are the salivary, mucous, protein and enzyme producing glands. *Plus!* The exocrine functions of your liver and pancreas add to their already long list of usefulness (like cleaning your blood and regulating your blood sugars) by secreting bile and pancreatic juices into your gastrointestinal tract as well.

The RESPIRATORY System

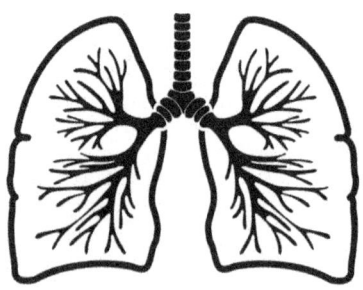

You can more or less happily last for about three weeks without food. Stagger on for about three days without water. But without oxygen? I wouldn't rate your chances after three minutes! After that, your brain begins to die no matter how much yoga breathing you've done. And sadly, the damage is pretty much irreversible even if you do manage to be revived or suck in some oxygen from somewhere. Or get back inside the spaceship.

Which is why it's important to tone up your lung health by exercising, eating healthily and giving up the smokes. Because your beautiful, spongy, delicate lungs are the primary organs of your respiratory system, which is responsible for breathing in oxygen and breathing out poisonous-to-humans carbon dioxide so at least the trees can breathe easy (and release oxygen into the atmosphere for all those dependent upon it).

All being well, this exchange of gases – O2 in / CO2 out – goes on automatically. Day after day for as long as we live, oxygen from your lungs is moved into your bloodstream and carried around your body, refreshing and renewing everything it can reach. Then your red blood cells scoop up all the leftover carbon dioxide, transport it back to your lungs via your veins, you breathe it out and the whole process starts over again. Perhaps this automatic process is why we rarely think about the importance of our respiratory systems until we can't breathe satisfactorily at all.

You can help keep your respiratory system healthy with regular exercise, deep breathing, getting a good night's rest, eating a nutritious diet and keeping hydrated. And not smoking!

THE CARDIOVASCULAR (or CIRCULATORY) System

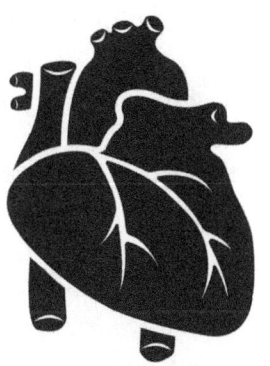

Your cardiovascular system consists of the heart, all the blood vessels in your body and your blood. Its main function is to carry oxygen and nutrients to the cells of your body and then carry wastes and deoxygenated blood away from the cells for recycling and disposal.

I've already briefly discussed the amazing muscle types of your heart and blood vessels in the sections on cardiac muscle and smooth muscle. But did you know that the amazingly constant muscular pumping action of your heart pushes the equivalent of more than 14,000 litres of blood around your body every day through five main types of blood vessels? Blood vessels form the living system of tubes that carry blood both to and from the heart. These hardworking muscular tubes are your arteries, arterioles, capillaries, venules and veins.

In the human body, there are more than 96,000 kilometres of blood vessels through which your heart pumps blood. That's about 60,000 miles if you don't do metric. About 40,000 kilometres (25,000 miles) of that is taken up by your capillaries, the smallest and most numerous blood vessels. Obviously, it's impossible to accurately count each and every one of them but – depending on your information source – you have between 300 million and 10 *billion* capillaries!

The blood vessels that take blood away from your heart are called arteries. The biggest artery in your body is one that comes out of your heart called the aorta. Smaller arteries branch off from the aorta and divide into smaller arteries the further away from the heart they go. The smallest arteries that that connect to the capillaries are called arterioles.

The blood vessels that return the used blood to the heart begin at the end of the capillaries and are called venules. Venules become larger as they proceed towards the heart and become veins. The two largest systemic veins in your body are called the vena cava. The inferior (which means 'below' in anatomical terms) vena cava takes blood from the lower half of your body back to your heart. The superior (which means 'above' in anatomical terms) vena cava takes blood from the upper part of your body back to the heart.

The circulation of your blood goes like this:

HEART → ARTERY → ARTERIOLE → CAPILLARY → VENULE → VEIN → HEART

There are two different circulations in your circulatory system – *systemic* and *pulmonary*. Systemic circulation is how the blood moves to most of your body. Pulmonary (meaning 'about the lungs' in anatomical terms) circulation is how deoxygenated blood goes through your lungs to absorb oxygen and release CO_2, and then the freshly *re*-oxygenated blood flows back to your heart.

You can help keep your heart healthy by exercising regularly, eating a nutritious diet, avoiding high fat processed foods, controlling your

cholesterol, managing and reducing stress levels, getting a good night's sleep and staying at a healthy weight. Oh, and no smoking!

The NERVOUS System

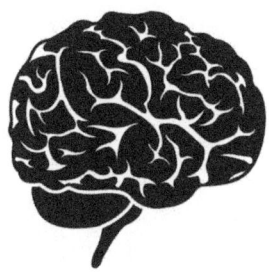

Your nervous system is responsible for the control of your body and the internal communication among its many parts and systems. It is made up by your brain and spinal cord (which together are called the central nervous system), your sensory organs (organs which allow you to see, hear, taste, smell, balance, etc.) and all the nerves that connect these organs with the rest of your body. Sensory receptors for the general senses like touch, temperature and pain are found throughout most of your body. All the sensory receptors in your body are connected to pathways that carry their sensory information to your central nervous system (CNS) 'command centre' to be processed and integrated.

The nervous system allows you to sense stimuli such as light, sound, smell and touch. It can send rapid communications within your body to communicate sensations such as pleasure, pain, illness, injury, heat and cold. It governs movement and balance. Allows perception, emotion, thought and rapid response to the environment. With such a huge workload, it's no surprise that your nervous system consumes as much as 25% of the kilojoules you eat to allow you to feel, think and respond.

The four main functions of your nervous system are:

- **Sensory** – detection of information from sensory signals about the internal and external conditions your body is experiencing

- **Communication** – reporting of sensory signals to the central nervous system

- **Integration** – processing of sensory information sent to the central nervous system for evaluation, interpretation, decision making, action, disposal or storage

- **Motor** – activation of bodily responses to commands from your central nervous system in smooth, skeletal or cardiac muscle and glandular tissues.

The part of your nervous system outside your brain and spinal cord is called the peripheral nervous system (or PNS for short). The PNS has two parts – the somatic (or voluntary) nervous system and the autonomic (or involuntary) nervous system.

The Somatic (or voluntary) nervous system controls both the voluntary movements and the reflex arcs of your skeletal muscles according to the information and impulses received from your sensory receptors. It is composed of two parts:

- **cranial nerves** – which carry nerve impulses in and out of the brain

- **spinal nerves** – which carry nerve impulses in and out of the spinal cord.

Your somatic nervous system is composed of two types of nerves – which are connected at the CNS by interneurons to facilitate 'two-way communication' traffic:

- **afferent neurons** – responsible for carrying messages from your sensory receptors to your 'central command' (CNS)

- **efferent neurons** – responsible for carrying messages from 'central command' to the effector organs.

THE 12 VITAL OPERATING SYSTEMS OF THE ANALOG BODY

In addition to controlling voluntary muscle movements, the somatic nervous system is involved in controlling involuntary muscle movements known as reflex arcs. You probably call them your reflexes.

The autonomic (or involuntary) nervous system functions automatically, keeping the smooth muscle of your heart, lungs, intestine, kidneys, blood vessels and your sweat, salivary and digestive glands ticking along without you having to think about it. Your autonomic nervous systems also controls your blood pressure, heartbeat, digestion, metabolism, body temperature, urination and *homeostasis*. The latter is your body's tendency to maintain its own stability in the face of environmental changes (for example, how your body tries to maintain an average temperature of 37 degrees Celsius or 98.6 degrees Fahrenheit, no matter what).

You can help keep your nervous system healthy by exercising regularly, reducing stress, getting a good night's sleep, avoiding processed foods and toxic chemicals (lead, arsenic, carbon monoxide, cigarettes, etcetera), eating a nutritious diet, monitoring your thyroid and blood sugar, staying hydrated and having regular check-ups.

The DIGESTIVE System

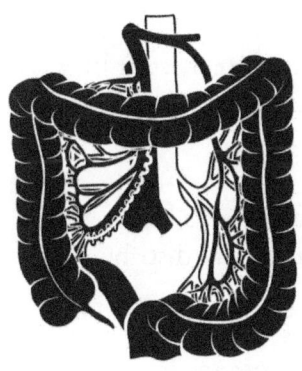

Who would have thought that series of hollow organs joined together in a long twisting tube from your mouth to your anus would become such a regular and compelling topic of public interest? Over the past decade the digestive system has become big news and big business. So, it's a good idea to have a working knowledge of yours – if only to keep up with what people are talking about (you'll find more information in Chapter 5).

Your digestive system is the group of organs that break down food to absorb nutrients. Most people think of their digestive tract as their stomach. However, your digestive system starts just inside your lips and includes your teeth, salivary glands, oral epithelium *and* your tongue! Outside the digestive 'tube', your liver, pancreas and gallbladder are also intricately involved in the processing of your food.

Here is the basic anatomy inside the 'tube' of your digestive system from beginning to end:

MOUTH ➜ OESOPHAGUS ➜ STOMACH ➜ SMALL INTESTINE ➜ LARGE INTESTINE ➜ COLON ➜ RECTUM ➜ ANUS

To process your food intake into useful nutrients for your body to use for nourishment, energy and repair, humans have six stages of food processing. Here's the simplified version of what happens:

1. **Ingestion** – taking food into your mouth

2. **Mechanical processing** – your teeth cut, tear and grind food into smaller pieces, your salivary glands add enzymes, mucous, antimicrobials and make food easy to swallow and your stomach churns and mixes ingested food

3. **Digestion** – chemical breakdown of food into small organic molecules of sugars and proteins suitable for absorption

4. **Secretion** – cells in your gastrointestinal tract, your liver, gallbladder and pancreas secrete water, enzymes, acids, buffers and salts to aid absorption

5. **Absorption** – the movement of micronutrients, water and vitamins into your blood and lymph vessels for distribution to your body's cells

6. **Excretion (defecation)** – the removal of wastes and indigestible substances.

THE 12 VITAL OPERATING SYSTEMS OF THE ANALOG BODY

You can help keep your digestive system healthy by getting plenty of exercise, reducing stress, getting a good night's sleep, eating a high fibre nutritious diet, incorporating pre and probiotics into your diet (see Chapter 5), limiting high fat and processed foods, choosing lean meats in smaller quantities, drinking water for hydration and avoiding overconsumption of caffeine and alcohol. Oh, and no smoking!

The REPRODUCTIVE System

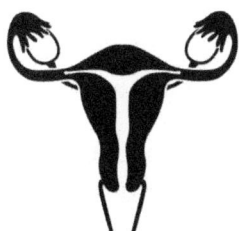

Generally speaking, human beings have two biological sexes – male and female. Plus, quite a lot of ambiguity in between. Hence, the fascinating and often confusing questions of nominal, neural, physical or psychological gender fluidities.

As with everything else in the *analog* world, we know there are many variations of normality. No matter how rare that normal variation may be. Nothing is predictably linear. Especially the distribution of chromosomes which determine sex – as opposed to 'gender'. In fact, these days, the term 'gender' is used broadly to classify a range of identities that don't necessarily correspond to either established cultural binary norms or other prevailing ideas of what constitutes male or female in terms of gender labels.

Even so, the term certainly doesn't explain the ever-increasing variations of DNA associated with chimerism – a rare condition – where people have been found to have two different blood types or even develop different sexual organs from those that might logically be associated with the rest of their body. Nor does the two sexes only normality theory explain people born intersex. That is, people born with any of several variations in sex characteristics, including chromosomes, gonads, sex hormones or genitals that, according to the UN Office of the High Commissioner for Human Rights, 'do not fit the typical definitions for male or female bodies'.

All of which can lead to all sorts of bewilderment, fear, alienation and identity trauma when people start talking about reproduction and there being *only two sexes*. As, indeed, there can be much debate, confusion and identity issues around accessing the reproductive system through in-vitro fertilisation (IVF), artificial insemination and surrogacy.

Much has been written about the sexual and reproductive organs of human females and males, so it would be superfluous to reproduce it here. Suffice to say, that if you are looking to reproduce there are certain reproductive requirements which cannot be denied. For the time being (at least) you will need to either have or have access to the following:

A female reproductive system which consists of:

- **Ovaries** – at least one of a possible two which produce ova (eggs) and female hormones

- **Fallopian tubes** – at least one of a possible two through which ova travel to reach your uterus

- **A uterus** – a muscular organ which (i) prepares for the possibility of a fetus every month and sheds its lining during menstruation when fertilisation doesn't occur or (ii) supports and nourishes implantation of a fertilised egg so that it can grow as a fetus over its 40-week development before birth via the vagina

- **A vagina** – the muscular tube leading from outside the female body to the cervix (or narrow passageway) which forms the lower end of the uterus.

A male reproductive system which will consist of:

- **Testes** – at least one of a possible two which manufacture sperm and male hormones

- **Vas deferens** – at least one of a possible two approximately 30cm thin tube known as the sperm ducts

- **Ducts and accessory glands** – involved in the transmission of sperm to the female via the penis

- **A penis** – with or without a protective foreskin covering (depending on parental or cultural choice at birth or shortly thereafter).

Always remember – with the odds of you being born at all running at about 1 in 400 trillion, you've already *won* the lottery by just making it this far! You're a living, breathing miracle of chance.

Needless to say though, you should prepare yourself for parenthood by improving your fitness levels, nutrition, sexual and general health because fertilisation, pregnancy, birth and child rearing are relentlessly analog in nature – requiring blood, sweat, tears, gumption, rat cunning, resolve and elbow grease.

The RENAL and URINARY EXCRETORY System

Your kidneys may seem of piddling importance in the scheme of things but just ask anyone who's ever been on dialysis how important they are. This system consists of your kidneys, ureters, bladder and urethra. Its function is to filter out excess fluid and other substances from your blood in the form of urine.

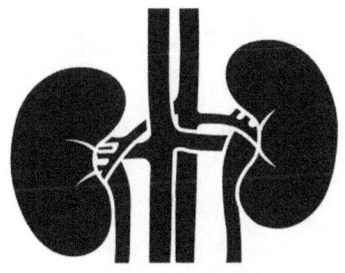

You have two bean-shaped kidneys, about 11cm in length, situated beneath the lower ribs of your back. Each kidney is attached to a ureter, a tube that carries excreted urine into your bladder and, from there, down the loo it goes.

Your kidneys may be small but they do a mammoth list of jobs – balancing and maintaining your body fluids; monitoring the levels of various chemicals, acids and electrolytes; filtering waste from food, medications and toxic substances; removing toxins; regulating your blood pressure; and creating hormones that help produce red blood cells and promote bone health.

A good indicator of how efficient your kidneys are at ridding you of toxins is the 2019 Australian Criminal Intelligence Commission's sixth 'National Wastewater Drug Monitoring Program' report. Based on wastewater data for August 2018, the report stated that more than 9.6 tonnes of methylamphetamine, 4 tonnes of cocaine, 1.1 tonnes of MDMA, and more than 700kg of heroin were consumed in Australia that year! Yep! It all washed down the loo, along with an avalanche of excreted food colourants, preservatives, bulking agents, flavour enhancers, vitamin supplements, fake raspberry cordial and a few thousand mobile phones.

You can help keep your kidneys healthy by exercising, controlling your blood sugar, monitoring your blood pressure, eating a nutritious diet and not smoking. And, yes, the best drink for the smooth function of your kidneys is WATER!

The ENDOCRINE System

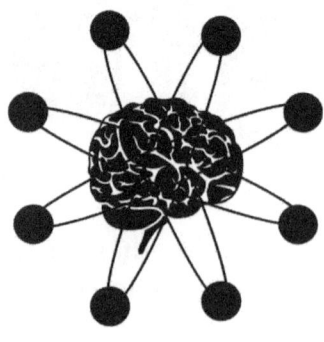

Simply put, your endocrine system is a work of art! A network of ductless glands that secrete chemicals called hormones into your blood to help your body functioning properly without you even knowing how damn tricky that is to execute. And all you need to do is stand back and appreciate the sheer genius of it.

THE 12 VITAL OPERATING SYSTEMS OF THE ANALOG BODY

Hormones are chemical messengers that coordinate and regulate a whole range of bodily functions and internal processes. These hormones act as chemical messengers for a large number of cells and tissues. In fact, almost every metabolic activity in your body is governed and integrated by hormones.

Unsurprisingly, most of the glands in your endocrine system are the main hormone producers in your body, such as the hypothalamus, pituitary, parathyroids, adrenal glands, reproductive glands, thyroid and pineal body. Although some other organs, such as your kidneys, liver, thymus, skin – and even your heart, lungs and brain – also produce hormones, which have work to do throughout your body.

For example, your digestive system and endocrine systems work neatly together, mostly through your pancreas, to produce and circulate digestive enzymes and hormones which tell your digestive system when to start and stop digesting food. Clever, huh?

Your endocrine system also works with your nervous system to organise and integrate signals from both your body and the environment. However, while your nervous system produces immediate effects, your endocrine system is comparably slower in its kick-off although it delivers a more prolonged effect in the end. Hormones like cortisol, produced by your adrenal glands during stress, can change both appetite and metabolic pathways in skeletal and smooth muscles for hours or even weeks after an intensely stressful event! (See Chapters 11 and 12 for tips on how to turn off your adrenal glands to relax or get a good night's sleep.)

The enormous 24/7 work of every ductless hormone secreting gland in your endocrine system would easily take a book of its own to do real justice to its importance. But as I said in the beginning of this chapter – this entire chapter is all just a taste so you can get back in touch with your body and appreciate the work it does even when you're sleeping.

You can help keep your endocrine system healthy by getting plenty of exercise, regular blood tests, reducing stress levels, getting a good night's sleep and eating a nutritious diet.

The LYMPHATIC System

Since when does the human body have *two circulatory systems*? Since some anatomical brainiac, trying to figure out how to explain the phenomenon of your lymphatic system, took a good long lateral thinking kind of look at how it cleverly runs alongside your cardiovascular system and twigged that the body actually has *TWO* 'circulatory systems', that's when.

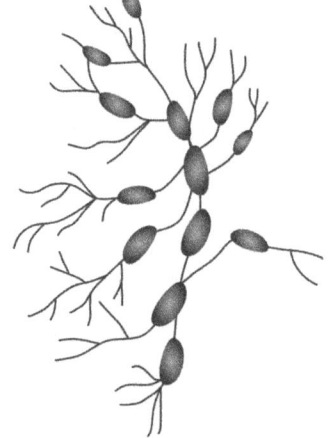

The lymphatic system works with the cardiovascular system to return body fluids to the blood. The lymphatic system is also an important part of your immune system which helps remove excess fluids, cellular debris, pathogens, proteins and bacteria from the tissues. Its primary function is to transport lymph, a fluid containing infection-fighting white blood cells throughout your body.

Your lymphatic system is composed of lymph nodes, lymph and lymphatic vessels. Lymph nodes filter the lymph, a clear sticky fluid that also bathes body cells and carries white blood cells which protect your body from viruses - as well as clearing away waste products.

Lymph nodes are located in groups throughout your body and are responsible for draining specific areas of your body. However, the largest node groupings are found in your neck, armpits and groin areas. Swollen lymph nodes in certain areas of your body may indicate that your body is dealing with infection or injury (or cancer) in that location or nearby.

In addition to nodes and vessels, major parts of the lymph tissue are located in the bone marrow and your:

- **thymus** – located in the neck above your heart. Its function is to generate lymphocytes which are white blood cells that help the immune system fight off illness.

- **tonsils** – small organs located in the back of your throat. You can see them as two lumps of tissue when you open your mouth wide. They help trap pathogens, such as bacteria or viruses that enter your mouth and contain immune cells that produce antibodies that kill these pathogens before they can spread to the rest of your body.

- **adenoids** – found in your upper nasal cavity and not easily seen. They help trap viruses and bacteria that enter your nose. Your adenoids are covered by a layer of mucus and hairlike structures called cilia, which help push nasal mucus down your throat and into your stomach.

- **spleen** – primarily associated with red blood cell turnover, it also clears bacteria and other pathogens that have been coated with antibodies.

- Your heart, lungs, intestines, liver and skin also contain lymphatic tissue.

Lymphatic tissue is vitally important for your immune system. If you didn't have a lymphatic system to drain away the excess fluid in your tissues it would build up and be very, very swollen and uncomfortable.

You can help keep your lymphatic system healthy with regular exercise (especially using a rebounder or mini trampoline which is also easy on the joints for older people or those with injuries), eating a varied and nutritious diet which includes lots of greens, herbs, fruit and other plant food, reducing stress, booking a massage, dry skin brushing and getting a good night's sleep.

The IMMUNE System

Last but by no means least is your immune system. The governor of your body's defences against infectious organisms and other invaders. Through a series of steps called 'the immune response' the immune system attacks organisms and substances that invade body systems and cause disease.

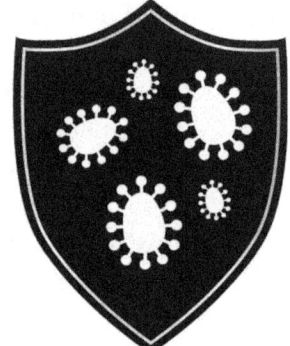

The key primary lymphoid organs of your immune system include your thymus and bone marrow - as well as secondary lymphatic tissues like your spleen, tonsils, lymph vessels, lymph nodes, adenoids, skin and liver. Your white blood cells are also part of your immune system.

As your first line of defence against disease, quite obviously, your lymphatic system and all of its tissues and fluids are vital components of your immune system, although the lymphatic system has other functions too and is part of the circulatory system as well as your immune system.

The human body has two major types of immunities – 'acquired' and 'innate'. Acquired immunity is associated with the lymphatic system and defined as specific or adaptive immunity. Innate immunity is natural or non-specific types of immunity present at birth and is not acquired via the lymphatic system.

Disorders of the immune system can result in autoimmune diseases, inflammatory diseases and cancer. Obviously, the bottom line is you really need your immune system, so you'd better look after it.

You can help keep your immune system healthy by regular exercise, eating plenty of fruits and vegetables, avoiding junk food and processed foods, cutting down on alcohol, reducing stress, getting enough sleep, keeping within a healthy weight range, washing your hands and keeping up with your vaccinations. I don't think I need

THE 12 VITAL OPERATING SYSTEMS OF THE ANALOG BODY

to remind you again that smoking doesn't work well for any of your body's systems at this point.

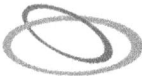

So, there you have it. YOU in a proverbial 'nutshell'. The real flesh and blood YOU! *Analog* to the core. No site access passwords. No remote controls. No offshore digital help centres. Just a miraculous conglomeration of mutually dependent *analog* systems that respond rather well to your tender loving care. If you care to pay attention.

CHAPTER 4

The Power of REAL food

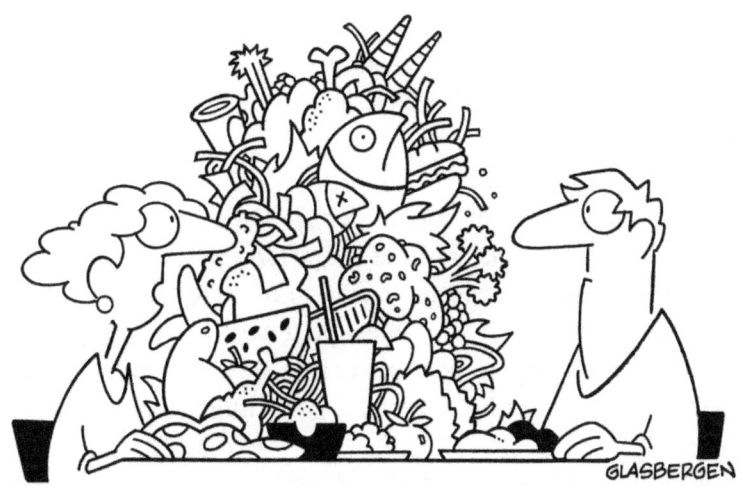

"I'm supposed to eat kale for smoother skin, turkey for stronger nails, fish for thinner thighs, oats for cardiovascular benefits, cabbage for leaner abdominals, salmon for softer hair, beets for a healthier colon, steak for muscle tone, blueberries for lower cholesterol, pasta for greater endurance, cheese for younger teeth and bones...."

How many times have you heard someone exclaim with righteous indignation – 'Noooooo! Surely not the (*fill in the blank*)! I thought (*fill in the blank*) was good for you!'

Surprisingly, it's arguably true that too much of *anything* – including the good stuff – is likely to kill you. However, there's also a fair chance that being constantly overwhelmed by wellness industry information bombarding us day in, day out, will eventually stress you out so entirely that your brain will just *snap*. Especially, if you're simply scanning, cherrypicking and talking about it, rather than actually applying any of it.

Over the last 150 years there have been gazillions of research reports, articles and books written about what's good for you and what's not.

What to eat for this and that. What's now officially declared poisonous. Real news and fake about the latest 'superfoods'. From the sublime to the ridiculous. The preposterous to the downright dangerous. However, it's only been in the last 20 odd years of the 'World Wide Web' that we've been inundated by it all. Millions of us, *googling* away 24/7. Fearful of missing out. Slaves to the algorithms.

Before that we had common sense. We grew things. We handpicked them. We cooked. We ate *real food*. We knew what we were eating and where it came from.

So, let's take another moment. Forget about trying to follow the dodgy and outdated US grain corporation's nutritional pyramids of last century. Take a deep breath and allow intermittent fasting, the Zen of Keto or whatever your latest plan is for an organic-vegetarian-dairy/sugar/gluten free sabbatical to just sit and fester for a while in the increasingly unsettled bowels of your mind.

> *'One thing I have long believed, and research agrees, is the mitochondrial-unfriendliness of the typical nutrient-poor American diet filled with sugar and processed, fried and hydrogenated oils. Bruce Ames, Ph.D., a respected molecular biologist and ageing expert at the University of California, regards the common nutrient deficiencies generated by the American diet as a profound cause of mitochondrial decay and accelerated ageing and disease. I've spoken with him in the past and he is right on the mark.'*
> **Dr. Stephen T Sinatra,**
> **cardiologist, bioenergetic psychotherapist &**
> **certified nutrition & anti-ageing specialist,**
> **from an online article 'What are Mitochondria?'**

Let's briefly explore how it is even possible that nutrition related, non-communicable diseases are on the rise in the wealthiest nations on earth. How health and longevity challenges – such as obesity, fatigue, migraines, chronic pain, food allergies, gastric reflux, diabetes, diverticular disease, metabolic syndrome, hypertension, cardiac disease, osteoporosis and gastrointestinal cancers – have risen exponentially in the past 30 years. The list goes on, of course, but don't forget depression and anxiety – which are both exacerbated by (you guessed it!) poor nutrition. Then consider, if you will, how we got to where we are now with our dispiriting lack of care for our fundamental daily nutrition.

Don't you find it odd that Australians live on the biggest fresh food producing island on earth and yet we lag only behind the USA with the second highest rate of non-communicable diet related illnesses on the planet? Over-nutrition. Under-nutrition. We've got it all.

The Chinese pay a premium for our fruits, vegetables, dairy and meats because they're so fresh and free of unregulated poisons. The Americans think we exist on a diet of barbequed lamb chops and prawns plucked from our pristine oceans and can't wait to get here to try them. The Japanese can't get enough of our Wagyu beef, abalone and ocean trout. The British clamour for our peaches, cherries, lamb and wine. India loves our chickpeas and lentils. Our fruits, nuts, vegetables, pork, cheeses, fish, seaweed and olives are in high demand out there in the big wide world. But what are *we* eating? Junk food.

Even with a daily choice of dozens of fabulously fresh options – some 97% of us simply can't be bothered chopping up some of this extraordinary fresh bounty for breakfast, lunch or dinner! Australians throw out a whopping eight billion dollars' worth of edible food weighing around four million tonnes every year! That's 345 kilos per household! Not only are we running out of places to safely put all this wasted and putrefying food, we're beginning to pay a hefty price for our laziness, complacency and sense of entitlement.

> *'Cooking is one of the strongest ceremonies for life. When recipes are put together, the kitchen is a chemical laboratory involving air, fire, water and the earth. This is what gives value to humans and elevates their spiritual qualities. If you take a frozen box and stick it in the microwave, you become connected to the factory.'*
>
> **Laura Esquivel, Mexican author**

For example, we grow at least the same variety of foodie wonderfulness as the Greeks, Italians and Turks do. But the main difference between us and them is they actually have a time-honoured cultural tradition of cooking and eating the stuff they grow on a daily basis. Which puts them at the top of the leader board among the healthiest eaters on the planet.

> *'Seriously? The Mediterranean diet? Tried that once. Too much effort. Lots of chopping? Meh. Why would you? Anyway, I've never liked vegetables…'*
> **One of my 'renovation clients' in their first session**

However, if you really can't see the point of all the chopping required of the many delicious versions of the Mediterranean diet (from Italy to Israel, Lebanon to Lisbon, etcetera) it's worth *googling* the 2015 study published by the Lancet Global Health Journal which looked at the diets of almost 4.5 billion adults across 167 countries. It found that although the worldwide consumption of healthy foods had increased over the previous 20 years, so had the intake of unhealthy foods, sugary drinks and processed foods. Alarmingly so. In fact, since the 1970s arrival and promotion of American junk food as the ubiquitous 'special treat', this particular trend has been slowly matched by the rising ill-health fallout experienced by its growing band of addicted consumers. You may also care to note that indigenous peoples worldwide have been some of the worst affected by their replacement of traditional *real food* with the Western World's limited diet and 'fast foods'. Big Food certainly has a case to answer here. No matter how much bleating they do about their menu of diabolically clever, food scientist formulated flavours and 'mouth-feels' being only for occasional use. The single point upon which I can agree with Big Food is that people are not *forced* to buy their products. Seduced, cajoled, addicted, hypnotised, yes. But not forced.

I should mention here that if you don't want to go Mediterranean, there's always the delicious varieties of real food served up by the Chinese, Vietnamese, Thais, South Americans, Mexicans, Africans, Sri Lankans and Indians. You will, however, still have to get to grips with chopping.

Which brings me to my next point. The enormous list of benefits to eating a wide variety of fresh foods. As opposed to unconsciously munching your way through the array of machined extrusions of denatured flour, sugar, chemicals and colourants somewhat ridiculously proclaimed as snacks, breakfast cereals, energy bars *et al*. Or the salt, sugar and fat laden Big Food franchise variations on chicken, the humble hamburger and their outrageous appropriations of the classic Italian pizza. Don't even get me started on the nutritional wastelands known as chicken nuggets and hot dogs!

> *'A vast body of research clearly demonstrates the health and anti-ageing benefits of a Mediterranean-type of diet, high in fruits and vegetables, which, in turn, are high in phytonutrient antioxidants. One study that particularly fascinated me identified hydroxytyrosol, a compound found in extra-virgin olive oil, as one of the most important phytonutrients in the Mediterranean Diet responsible for lowering the incidence of cardiovascular disease. The study, conducted by researchers at Shanghai's Institute for Nutritional Science, concluded that hydroxytyrosol stimulates the growth, development, and enhanced functionality of mitochondria.'*
>
> **Dr. Stephen T Sinatra,
> cardiologist, bioenergetic psychotherapist &
> certified nutrition & anti-ageing specialist**

Chopping up lots of different kinds of fresh foods and throwing them either raw into a bowl or tossing them about in a hot pan for your daily consumption is *key* to your health. And frankly, if you can't be doing with gathering and preparing fresh ingredients, herbs, spices, natural oils and nurturing your own creativity by cooking for yourself and your loved ones – where does that leave you? Up the nutritional creek, that's where. Because you've inadvertently absorbed the marketing message – that the cool crowd order in or eat out. That seductive aspirational marketing potion that keeps telling you that people who are really successful don't have to bother with learning how to cook because they can afford to outsource it. In the last two or three years there are even apps to 'help' you avoid cooking. The unconscious absorption of marketed trends is the most modern form of osmosis there is. Trouble is, it will not nourish you.

> 'Poor eating habits start at an early age. A lot of people don't get introduced to vegetables as children, and, therefore, never like them. Also, we are stuffing our faces with lots of carbohydrate junk, so we never get hungry.'
>
> **Dr Michael Mosley,**
> **medical journalist & health documentary maker**

As a 'people renovator', I spend a lot of time talking to my clients about the important role of nutrition in their general wellness, skin conditions, digestive problems, weight gain and pain management. And that includes clients referred to me for 'self-care' by other health professionals, especially those with anxiety, bipolar disorder and depression. I have yet to meet a client whose condition or energy levels cannot be improved by overhauling their daily nutrition to include vastly more variety. Asking them to keep a food diary for two weeks to see what they're really eating on a daily basis is both confronting and illuminating. Mainly because of the astonishingly small number of food types (therefor nutrients and complex fuels) the person sitting in front of me is actually running on. By the time I've counted white flour, sugar, caffeine and a splash of milk, often there are only two or three other items of any nutritional value. Frankly, it's a marvel how much punishment the human body can take. I'm staggered they're functioning at all!

> '... if you drink much from a bottle marked "poison", it is almost certain to disagree with you, sooner or later.'
>
> **Alice, *Alice in Wonderland* by Lewis Carroll**

There are those who've lost the will to cook. Those who don't even know how to cook. And the self-fulfilling prophesies who are addicted to the very foods making them feel awful in the first place.

These are some of the reasons I invented my **21 Foods a Day Plan**. It's not a diet as such. More like a life-altering challenge that also brings the opportunity to develop chef-like chopping skills. And, when you combine it with gentle exercise, massage and relaxation, it's dynamite! Certainly, one of the best ways I know to get people on the road to better health.

Let me give you some examples.

Maureen, 27, was referred to me by her psychiatrist. The psychiatrist had referred several of her patients to me over the years in the hope they would learn to take better care of themselves. My holistic approach to self-care and the creation of a personally tailored plan had worked well for her patients in the past. As usual, the brief was fairly open – apply all the tools at my disposal, one at a time, or in combination, to encourage Maureen to start taking her health seriously.

Diagnosed and treated for bipolar disorder for several years, Maureen was relatively stable on her medications. She was, however, utterly exhausted from morning till night, often very 'flat' of mood and the first signs of metabolic syndrome were appearing in her blood tests. She was on her way to type 2 diabetes. Her skin was dull. She was moderately overweight. A mere five minutes of moderate exercise on the rebounder to test her aerobic capacity was more than enough even though her heart rate didn't exceed 100 beats a minute. Tellingly, at the end of the first two weeks, her food diary revealed she ate breakfast, lunch and dinner at a certain burger franchise every day!

Shocking, I know. Although, I was heartened by her meticulous food and exercise record keeping on a shiny new iPad. Basically, she did no more exercise than walking short distances to and from her car. She ate the same five foods - bun, fries, mince patty, a slice each of tomato and pickle – three times a day. Sometimes four if she was particularly hungry, which she often was. If she was caught short, a couple of chocolate bars filled the gap. She was also constipated, 'farty' and often felt a bit nauseated. To top it off, she didn't cook and had little interest in learning how to. When I mentioned the 21 Foods a Day

Plan, she looked genuinely incredulous. That young woman really *loved* her burgers for two good reasons. They were convenient and tasty. The only thing to do was tackle the problem one burger at a time.

I was also going to have to somehow sweet-talk her into tapping some basic cooking skills notes into the iPad. First, I nutted out a shopping list for her which would last the entire first week. Then the breakfast burger went: replaced by a tastier homemade alternative – my 'deluxe eight to 10 ingredient chicken, meat or egg sandwich on wholegrain sourdough'. A simple enough concoction with built-in versatility, mouth-feel and tastiness.

The following week the shopping list became slightly longer. I taught her how to make a frittata – that yummy Italian hybrid of quiche and omelette which changes depending what leftovers you have or what's in the refrigerator or pantry. Then the lunch burger disappeared: replaced by a large slice of five vegetable frittata, accompanied by a salad of greens, olives, tomato, red onion, peas, grated carrot, a sprinkling of *dukkha*, finely chopped celery dressed with olive oil and fresh lemon juice.

Finally, the dinner burger went the way of all the others. Maureen had invested in a slow cooker by then. The shopping list had grown but was still manageable. I taught her how to make tasty casseroles and slow oven bakes of eight or so different ingredients. How to freeze and label the leftovers so she didn't have to cook every night. How to bake or mash sweet potato and steam some beans to go with it. How to toss mushrooms and herbs with olive oil in a pan and sprinkle them on salads or mash. All simple ways to increase nutritional uptake and avoid junky temptation.

Within six weeks she was eating close to 30 foods a day and she looked like a different person. Her eyes were clear. Her skin glowing. She was amazed by how much energy she'd recovered in such a short time. Her mood was considerably improved. She no longer felt like her 'head would explode' when she was hungry. And she'd slimmed down.

THE POWER OF REAL FOOD

'The food you eat can either be the safest and most powerful form of medicine... or the slowest form of poison.'
**Ann Wigmore,
holistic health practitioner & raw food advocate**

Jacquie was another kettle of fish, entirely. Although, she too was down to about three different foods a day. A slab of cheddar. A box of Jatz biscuits. The milk in her many cappuccinos. A high-flying executive in her early 50s, she first came to see me for relaxation, massage and self-care precipitated by the appearance of multiple lumps in her breasts. The first thing I did was book her an appointment with my breast cancer physician. Weeks of high stress and soul searching went by as she had one test after another. Happily, for Jacquie, the breast lumps eventually turned out to be cysts.

One day, during a soothing aromatherapy session, she asked me what she could do to improve her energy levels. She wondered if her diet had anything to do with her tendency towards cysts and extreme constipation. As we talked, it became apparent she ate neither breakfast nor lunch, running on empty for most of her days. Then she'd rush home from work to cook a beautiful meal for her husband and son and be so hungry she'd sink a couple of glasses of wine, a box of Jatz and a hefty slab of cheese while making it. Her self-imposed penance was to eat nothing for dinner. When I asked her why, she told me her weight had once ballooned to around 140 kilos after a difficult business partnership. Gastric band surgery had helped her lose about 80 kilos. She never wanted to put that weight on again, but she was definitely caught in a cycle of nutritional self-destruction.

Needless to say, she was highly doubtful that she could maintain her weight while adding 21 different foods a day to her diet. Fortunately, the upside of her breast cancer scare meant she was galvanised into taking some sort of action to improve her overall health. After some trial and error, what worked for her was to whip up a couple of boxes of what

I call 'nibbling salads' – one savoury, one sweet but both with protein and crunchy stuff. Between us we concocted many different versions of my 'eight to 10 ingredient salad' and my 'eight to 10 ingredient fruit salad'. Food she could graze on and pick at during the day. A staggered nutrition strategy to prevent her falling back into the 'eat anything really fast to stave off the low blood sugar' cycle.

When after a month she'd stopped cramming Jatz and cheese, was eating at least 21 different foods a day and hadn't put on any unwanted weight, she was thrilled. Six months later, she sent me a Christmas card thanking me for reigniting her love of food and cooking and telling me how much better she felt now that she was eating properly.

Barbara was a retired teacher in her late 50s. Approaching her 60th birthday, she already suffered from three of Australia's most common non-communicable and preventable diseases. Her blood pressure was high. About 160cms tall, she was a chunky 20 kilos over her ideal weight and already medicated for type 2 diabetes.

Her GP had been suggesting regular exercise for years, but Barbara was always too busy to schedule it in. It was only when she retired and wanted to go travelling that she bravely picked me out from the thousands of personal trainers listed online in Sydney because I advertised that I trained older people *'to do what you've always wanted to do'*. It was a good move. She couldn't bear the idea of 'prancing about in a gym'. After years of neglecting her own health as she looked after others, she needed lots of one-on-one encouragement to get moving again. She also needed someone who could teach proper low impact exercise form, so she didn't injure herself. Which would have put the kibosh on her international travel dreams before she'd even set off.

As weight loss was a primary concern, we started with the food diary. Although she'd left the temptations of the staff tearoom for several months, morning and afternoon tea breaks with processed biscuits and cake were still a daily habit. In fact, now that she wasn't rushing between classrooms, she'd even put on several kilos since she'd retired. I had to put it to her gently that I didn't consider biscuits and cake to be actual food. Certainly, they were not included in the 21 Foods a Day Plan as *actual* food. To make matters worse, the rest of her daily meals were almost entirely processed and devoid of nutrition. Toast and tea for breakfast. Toasted ham and cheese sandwich for lunch. A chop and frozen beans and fries for dinner. Dessert was ice cream and more cake. Far too much salt, sugar and empty calories, for sure. And where was the nourishment to repair her ageing body? The best I could say was at least she was never hungry. Nevertheless, it was plain to see she wasn't absorbing anything that might sustain her either.

So, where did we start? Because there's nothing worse than changing your diet *and* being left hungry, I'm a great believer in adding more food. To start her on the path to 21 different foods a day we started gradually adding *fresh* foods to what she was already eating. For example – instead of toast and jam, multigrain toast with avocado, ricotta, tomato, sprouts and poached egg was added to breakfast. A home packed roll stuffed with eight different vegetables and protein and a cup of homemade vegetable soup was added to lunch. Fish, chicken, steam-ups, salads and stir fries were added to dinner. Apples and bananas dipped in LSA (a delicious ground nutty meal made from linseeds, almonds and sunflower seeds) took the place of cakes and biscuits. Yoghurt and berries became dessert.

During that time, as well as her twice weekly strength and aerobic classes with me, I insisted she walk every day (with at least one difficult hill) for at least 30 - 40 minutes. We built up to that slowly over a period of several months in the same slow steady way we gradually added real food to her diet. Ironing out problems, likes and dislikes along the way until she had a customised routine she could really call her own. Once a week, on a day of her choosing, she could forget about her regular daily walk. She could even opt for a piece of seriously good cake! Not a sugar hit. Not a habit. Not just eating it because everyone else was. Nope. Something she really could enjoy. A high-quality temptation worth temporarily falling off the wagon for.

A year later, she was 22 kilos lighter, her blood pressure medication was reduced, she was free of type 2 diabetes and off to Europe.

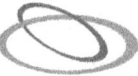

'The food and beverages we consume (our diet) play an important role in our overall health and wellbeing. Food provides energy, nutrients and other components that, if consumed in insufficient or excess amounts, can result in ill health. A healthy diet helps to prevent and manage health risk factors such as overweight and obesity, high blood pressure and high cholesterol, as well as associated chronic conditions, including type 2 diabetes, cardiovascular disease and some forms of cancer. Diet-related chronic conditions are among the leading causes of death and disability in Australia.'
Australian Institute of Health & Welfare report 2018

CHAPTER 5

When the Food Leaves the Fork: My '3 Golden Rules' & Other Stories

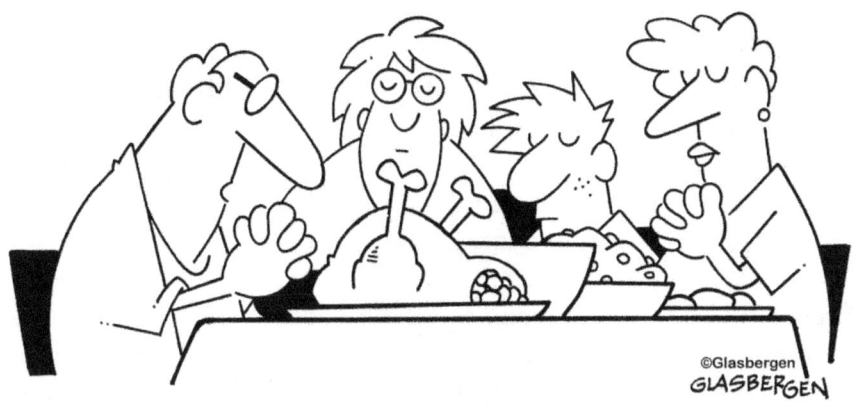

"Lord, make us grateful for the cholesterol, diabetes, high blood pressure, weight gain and indigestion we are about to receive."

To my mind, the digestive tract is the great leveller. Never mind who you *think* you are – or how important, rich, poor, brilliant or dimwitted – you are, essentially, an approximately nine metre *tube*. And, in the way of tubes, the story goes like this:

stuff goes in one end ➔ tumbles about ➔ and eventually comes out the other end

I call this my 'theory of digestion for eight to nine-year-olds' because, unlike grown-ups, they already understand that we are all fundamentally the same and are not bothered by the subject of pooing.

Also, because it appears that (with the possible exception of gastroenterologists) only eight to nine-year-olds find the entire end-to-end business of digestion captivating enough to be worthy of close attention. They certainly understand how rollickingly amusing the processes can be. Especially the hilarious phenomena of burping, farting and pooping. Fortunately, they are too young to understand what can happen when you take your inner tube and its functions for granted.

Enough, already? You may be reading this while bolting your lunch. Trying to drift off to sleep after a long, tough day and a big late dinner. Browsing your phone on the loo to distract yourself from chronic constipation. Swallowing antacids as you read this chapter while waiting in some dingy corridor for exam, job or court case results. One way or another, you may be in no state to get to grips with the machinations of your inner tube. Fine. Apologies. Let's try something less confronting. More glamorous, even…

Scene #1: Head to toe in sequins, you sit in a fancy restaurant. Hungry as. A waiter is walking past you with a wafting, sizzling platter of deliciousness. It's not your order but behind your perfect lip gloss your salivary glands are kick-starting the digestive process anyway. Your mouth begins to water…
~ This response is known as 'the conditioned salivary reflex'.

Scene #2: It's your first public performance of *Nessun Dorma*. The curtain rises. Mist envelops the stage. The overture begins. Your stomach seems suddenly full of butterflies as you realise your faultless Italian has been totally hijacked and obliterated by the English translation you learned for expression. 'None shall sleep… none shall sleep…' The butterflies turn to lead…
~ The butterflies and leaden responses signal your 'enteric nervous system' is trying to tell you something about your situation.

Scene #3: You arrive at Mount Everest base camp moments before a blizzard, bursting for the heavy-duty latrine from something you ate last night. An announcement from the Nepalese Government is

delivered over the loudspeaker by your tour guide – i.e. from here on up, you are required to make arrangements to carry your faeces with you. The Sherpas heave a sigh of relief that *they* will no longer have to remove close to 12,000 kg of human excrement from Everest every climbing season. (True story!)
~ Your gobsmacked response reveals much about how unprepared, inconvenienced or outraged you are. It's also a good indicator of how much thought you've ever given to the logistics surrounding the daily end product of your digestive system.

Makes you think doesn't it? How dependent are we on the profound daily work of our digestive system? The sheer *mashability* of it! ('Mashable' – two or more online applications that work together and/or within each other.) And how much of it we simply take for granted – workability, absorbability, reliability, regularity, controllability *et al*. Hardly anyone spares a thought for the real daily grind of our digestive systems. Peristalsis – the automatic food churning process of the smooth muscle of our digestive tracts that further pulverises our chewed food into tiny particles so we can extract life-enhancing nutrients. The automatic provision of enzymes, hormones and other chemicals to assist with absorption. Organising the storage and gradual usage of nutrients and sending the rest off down the tract for elimination. How the gut's 'second brain' – the enteric nervous system – influences our mood and wellbeing. And how much we take the convenience of modern toilets for granted. Out of sight, out of mind is pretty much how most people over the age of eight consider the riveting, life affirming miracle of it all.

All that functionality and nutrition aside for the moment, there are other important reasons why you need to take care of your digestive tract and what you put into it. For example, your gut plays a vital role in many other areas of your health, including your immune system, daily headspace and ability to ward off depression. It may surprise you to know that about 80% of your immune system is located in your gut! And something like 95% of your serotonin – the 'feel good' neurotransmitter – is produced in your bowels! In fact, altered levels of peripheral serotonin have been linked to irritable bowel syndrome (IBS), cardiovascular disease and osteoporosis as well.

Did you know, for example, that even if you're just experiencing what you may consider common 'garden variety' gastrointestinal problems you may be suffering from an unhealthy gut? And that same unhealthy gut can be headed down the path of the new wave of non-communicable lifestyle diseases already plaguing the planet? We all know *someone* suffering in silence (or otherwise) from acid reflux, heartburn, gut pain, wind, irritable bowel syndrome (IBS), colitis, constipation or diarrhoea. In fact, the more junk we eat, the more stressed out we become, the more over-the-counter drugs we swallow to keep symptoms at bay, the more these problems are increasing in the community. And the news that bowel cancer is now the most common internal cancer in Australia with mortality second only to lung cancer is disturbing to say the least. But did you know that gut problems tackled early are often both preventable and reversible? You just have to have the 'guts' to get on to it, pronto.

According to The Gut Foundation of Australia:

> *'Half the population complain of some digestive problem in any 12-month period.*
>
> *The key to preventing and even reversing these problems is to change our views on healthy eating and lifestyle. This does not mean boring hideous or stodgy special diets... Our educational and medical efforts focus on primary prevention with recommended dietary changes for all of us, from an early age, towards a diet with more natural fibre and less fats and sugars. We strongly emphasise a diet with a wide variety of fruits and vegetables, grains and cereals and delicious ways to prepare and enjoy them! What is there to lose? And you will gain better health, more energy and the bonus of fewer or no gut problems.'*

The problem is, that few people (with rare but notable exceptions) like to talk about what's going on in their gut. Sometimes, it's embarrassment. Sometimes, to avoid scrutiny of their daily intake of food and drink. Sometimes, because the problem has been going on for so long that it seems normal and therefor unremarkable. And sometimes, because discussing the texture of your poo, the intensity of your windiness (at either end) or chronic indigestion seems like undignified bellyaching and therefor distasteful.

There are many books written about digestion and the health of the human digestive tract and at the end of this book, I'll list a few of them for your further reading. But, for the moment, let's assume you're regularly eating a virtual rainbow of fresh fruit and vegetables, with healthy whole grains, nuts and seeds, cold-pressed oils, beans and greens and lentils, oily fish, small amounts of meat (or none at all), cultured and fermented foods rich in probiotics and prebiotics and plenty of fresh water. And now, *tah dah!* to head off some of the most basic digestive problems, let's look at **My Three Golden Rules to Aid Digestion** when your food leaves your fork:

(1) **Slow down:** this means loading *small* amounts of food on your fork and putting your fork down between mouthfuls.

(2) **Chew, chew, chew and chew some more:** the last thing your long-suffering stomach needs is un-chewed food landing in it in great stodgy, indigestion triggering lumps! If you make sure you choose food that needs to be chewed (i.e. fresh food with soluble and insoluble fibre, rather than processed pap) the chewing should come naturally and the friendly bacteria and cilia in your gut will love you right back because they'll be able to do their job properly.

(3) **Avoid overeating:** everyone knows that bloated, concrete-in-the gut feeling. However, if you follow the first two rules, this third one should be a cinch because you'll actually receive the 'full' message from your sensible gut 'brain' long before you've overeaten.

Forks piled choc-a-block. Mouths filled to bursting. Barely a moment between mouthfuls. Stress much? Most of us are in such a screaming hurry to get food into ourselves that we bolt it down the hatch, scarcely chewing or tasting it at all. Is it any wonder that our poor confused digestive systems often repay our disregard with belching, bellyache and borborygmi? And what, pray tell, is borborygmi? *Normal* borborygmi are simply the growlings and rumblings of your stomach. However, *abnormal* borborygmi are associated with crampy abdominal pain and stronger contractions of the intestinal muscle caused by increased gut distension due to additional amounts of trapped gases. Natural remedies include – water; eating something; chewing slowly; limited sugar, alcohol and acidic foods; avoiding gaseous drinks; discovering food intolerances; portion control; exercise and an active lifestyle.

When you come to think of it, it's an absolute marvel that the first two parts of your digestive system to tackle your food are your saliva and your teeth. Definitely a major reason to take good care of your teeth for as long as possible. Although we secrete saliva 24/7 at a rate of about 1 to 1.5 litres per day, when we begin to chew, the amount of saliva increases to act as a lubricant making your food easier to swallow. Saliva contains a raft of useful chemicals, salivary proteins, free amino acids and starch dissolving enzymes. It also helps to dissolve elements in your food to activate your pleasure-seeking tastebuds. The more thoroughly you chew your food, the more saliva you produce to render it ready to hit your stomach, the better your digestive system likes it.

FAQs

Is bloating normal?

Bloating is common after eating. You can avoid it by – chewing slowly and thoroughly; putting your fork down between mouthfuls; avoiding carbonated drinks while eating; going for a walk after dinner; avoiding certain trigger foods such as beans, lentils, split peas, cabbage, brussels sprouts; becoming aware of food intolerances; and avoiding high fat foods.

Definitely see your doctor for a check-up if bloating is becoming an uncomfortable everyday occurrence after most meals; or is accompanied by nausea, abdominal pain, constipation, diarrhoea, fatigue, unexpected weight loss or skin irritation.

What about wind?

As a general rule of thumb, you can tell which part of your gut is struggling by where the wind is coming from. If you're belching more than normal, it could be that you're eating too fast; are stressed; too talkative while eating and swallowing air; not chewing thoroughly; have a food or fizzy drink intolerance; a hiatus hernia; or a small intestine infection. If flatulence is your problem, consider a course of probiotics to rebalance your friendly gut bacteria (especially after treatment with antibiotics); lifestyle and dietary changes may be required; a brisk walk after dinner can often settle the problem *and* get you outside. As with bloating, if you've taken all the above into account and you're still windy, embarrassed and uncomfortable after every meal, it's time to see your doctor for a check-up. Don't just forget about it, okay? That's asking for trouble.

What is a food intolerance?

Seems like every man and his dog has a food intolerance these days. I'm not entirely sure *why* this is, but in most cases it's real and can be easily remedied. Firstly, a food intolerance is completely different from a food allergy. A food allergy triggers the immune system, while a food intolerance does not. A food allergy can prove extremely dangerous to health, while the worst manifestations of food intolerance are varied and usually more irritating and uncomfortable than life threatening. Symptoms of food intolerance can include bloating, cough, migraine, headaches, stomach-ache, runny nose, sinus pain, hives, feeling 'flu-ish' and diarrhoea; as well as aggravation of conditions such as asthma, eczema and psoriasis.

Although identifying food intolerances can take a long time, I find it useful to keep a food diary, back-dated at least three days before the onset of troublesome symptoms. This is because the onset of some food intolerances can take hours or several days and may persist for hours or days, depending on the sensitivity to the food and the amount consumed. But food diaries can definitely help pinpoint the culprits.

Common types of food intolerance are – lactose, wheat, grains in general, gluten, caffeine, and histamines present in mushrooms, pickles and cured foods. Other foods it may help you to avoid are sugary drinks, cakes, lollies, spicy foods with lots of chillies, and fried and processed foods. Finally, consider this – if there is a food you constantly crave and cannot live without, chances are you have an intolerance to it! Sad but true, as I'll explain in one of my case studies in this chapter.

How do you know if a processed food is going to cause a sensitivity problem?

Although natural fresh foods can also trigger sensitivities in susceptible people, it seems to me that diets high in processed, chemical and colourant laden foods are more often implicated in food sensitivities. Removing most (or *all* of them) from the diet is often key to recovery from annoying symptoms like cough, hives, reflux, bloating, sneezing, sinusitis, etcetera. When total avoidance isn't possible, I always tell my clients to at least keep consumption to a minimum and supplemented by fresh foods. Read food labels carefully. Pick the products with the least chemical names and numbers. And look out for vague 'weasel words' like 'spices', 'flavourings', 'preservatives added' which define nothing. Ingredients are labelled from the highest content to the lowest. So if, say, you're buying a nut bar and nuts are listed far down the line of ingredients or are the only recognisable food name (other than sugar) amongst several ingredients with long chemical names – just put it back on the shelf and find something more natural. Our digestive systems and livers take enough punishment from what we ingest and what's in our environment as it is without voluntarily consuming more unnecessary chemicals. Given that we have the same livers and digestive systems we had 5,000 or 10,000 years ago, and the regular consumption of chemical laden foods has been going on for a mere 50 years at best, it's unlikely our digestions have evolved sufficiently to deal with all the gut irritating additives. It's enough to make you break out in a rash just thinking about it!

Is water good for digestion?

Water is wonderful for pretty much every function of your body. In the digestive system it moistens food, helps dissolve nutrients, encourages the passage of food and waste through the digestive tract, helps soften your stools and reduces constipation and bloating. On the other hand, quenching your thirst by substituting fizzy, sweetened drinks, coffee and tea for pure water will irritate your gut, put you at risk of type 2 diabetes and make you age faster. Don't like the taste? Get over yourself. Water has no taste (unless you have the misfortune to live somewhere the water is tainted, in which case, attach a water purifying filter to your drinking water tap or boil your water first and stand it overnight in the fridge). Just a pure refreshing sensation.

Are probiotics really necessary? Why prebiotics? Who should I talk to about them?

The basic idea of probiotics for your digestion has been around for thousands of years. Probiotics are live bacteria and yeasts that are good for your digestive system. Although your body is full of both 'good' and 'bad' bacteria, essentially, 'bad' bacteria only become a problem when they outnumber the 'good' bacteria. Good bacteria are your body's natural probiotics and they live mostly in your colon working to strengthen your digestive tract and also prevent allergies and sensitivities to foods and other irritants. An intestinal tract that has an optimal balance of naturally occurring 'good' or 'friendly' bacteria is generally considered healthy. It's all to do with the balance.

An overgrowth of bad bacteria can be caused by – diets high in refined sugar, antibiotics, excessive amounts of alcohol, chronic stress, and diets low in fibre and essential nutrients.

There are three ways of restoring the balance of good bacteria in your gut:

- **a diet high in foods which are a rich source of probiotics** – cultured yoghurt, apple cider vinegar, 'kosher' lactic acid fermented dill pickles, kombucha, kimchi, coconut kefir and sauerkraut

- **prescribed probiotic cultures which come in capsules and pill form** – are specially formulated 'friendly' bacteria combinations formulated to address specific serious health problems, prescribed by doctors, naturopaths and other natural therapy practitioners to restore gut health after illness and antibiotic use

- **over-the-counter general probiotics** – in pill or capsule form sold by pharmacies for everyday gut health and minor maladies.

Although *prebiotics* and *probiotics* may sound the same, they are entirely different. Probiotics are a general term for friendly bacteria that live in your gut and you can add them to your gut via probiotic rich foods and prescribed combinations.

Prebiotics, on the other hand, are the nutritious fibre nutrients that feed your 'good' bacteria. That is, the plant-based fibres you consume when you eat a wide and varied diet of fruits, vegetables, nut and seeds. In short, it's the *prebiotics* that feed your probiotics. So vital to the whole process.

How does exercise affect the digestive system?

I'll talk more about the wonderful benefits of movement and exercise in Chapter 9. Briefly, regular cardiovascular exercise helps strengthen abdominal muscles and reduce stress levels. Exercise is known to reduce bowel sluggishness by stimulating intestinal muscles to push digestive contents through the digestive system. Walking, swimming, cycling, ballroom dancing are all fun ways to get your bowels moving. Who knew?

Why does my digestion play up when I'm stressed?

Stress affects the nerves of the digestive system and therefor can upset the intricate balance of your digestion. In some people, stress slows the digestive process causing bloating, pain, constipation or diarrhoea. Stress can also worsen conditions such as peptic ulcers, irritable bowel syndrome and Crohn's disease. It's worth mentioning here that chronic stress often goes hand-in-hand with erratic and comfort eating, poor food choices, high alcohol consumption and many more stressed-based habits that undermine your health. See Chapter 11 for some ideas on how to relax.

The following are examples of digestive problems solved with a few simple tweaks…

Some years ago, on a group tour to China, I was struck by how many Australians on the tour ate little or no vegetable matter and headed straight for the deep-fried dishes. Although I did my best not to waste a single vegetable dish (and there were some beauties, let me tell you), it seemed I was one of the few. One morning as I savoured my delicious Chinese scrambled eggs with tomato and spring onion with a side of fresh orange segments, a pallid middle-aged couple joined me at the table. Two of the most prolific eaters of the fried foods served at lunch and dinner, their plates were now piled high with Rice Crispies, white toast and what appeared to be dozens of those dinky single serve containers of jam and butter.

'You can have some too,' the wife answered my raised eyebrow. 'Foodwise, we're Chinesed out. Got the guide to send to Beijing for some *real* breakfast food.' Considering we were staying in a traditional Chinese country hotel, at the top of a mountain in Wudang Province, ferrying in white bread and Rice Krispies from the capital several hundred kilometres away was some feat, I said. But she didn't want to talk about that. She'd discovered I was an allied health professional and she wanted to talk about the state of her bowels. The constipation was crippling, she told me. Days without a movement. Just like at home, sometimes. She was so bloated she felt like she might explode, in fact. Did I have any remedies with me? Could I help? To cut her long story short, I recommended she eat only vegetables, a little steamed chicken and fruit for a few days, cut out all starch and fried stuff and start drinking water. With that, I finished my breakfast and made myself scarce. For several days, in fact. Until one day, as I wandered around the martial arts training compound of Shaolin, she found me again. And what a revelation! The pallid complexion was gone, her eyes were bright, and she couldn't wait to update me on the state of her bowels.

'*Who knew* a few vegetables and some water could fix everything?!' she said, looking truly incredulous.

Connie came to see me in the hope that some lymphatic drainage sessions might help reduce her chronic migraines. A vivacious Italian woman in her late forties, she'd found herself poleaxed by two or three migraines a week, a situation which required whole days in a darkened room and increasingly heavy-duty medication. Scans revealed nothing sinister and her doctors were at a loss to explain her worsening symptoms. I suggested she book in for a weekly combination massage of aromatherapy and neuromuscular massage to relieve the tension in her neck, shoulders and scalp. I then asked her to keep a 'food & mood' diary in between sessions. I also suggested she discuss with her doctor the possibility of a magnesium supplement as, according to the Australian Migraine Association, migraines are often a sign of chronic magnesium deficiency.

By the second week of massage treatment I had a clear idea of where her tensions lay – neck, shoulders, scalp, jaw, chest and solar plexus. But it was when she returned with the food diary that the role her digestive system was playing in her migraines showed up. Two big weeks of cooking and planning for the generous Italian traditions of entertaining around a wedding, a christening and an elderly birthday told me what I needed to know. Almost every major classic trigger for migraines was present – red wine, chocolate, coffee, oranges, tiramisu, cured meats, cheeses, eggplant, capsicums, tomatoes etcetera – exacerbated by the crushing stress that went with pulling off each occasion perfectly. She was stunned that neither her GP nor her neurologist had spoken to her about either magnesium or her diet. But by this stage, she thought the magnesium was starting to help her sleep slightly better, as well as taking the edge off her headaches. So, when I suggested she take the next step and avoid the classic Italian antipasto foods herself and gave her some alternative antipasto ideas which she liked, she was enthusiastic.

After three months of relaxing scalp, head, neck and shoulder massage with analgesic essential oils, a dietary change to avoid the migraine triggers and ongoing magnesium supplementation, Connie had reduced both her medication and the severity of her migraines, and was down to a single migraine episode every two to three weeks. Then she stopped coming. A wistful email thanked me for my assistance but explained that she could no longer eat differently from her family and had decided to go back on full strength medication.

I should like to add here that, while I appreciate the need to fit in with everyone else, especially family, it's important to follow your own path when it comes to ill health caused by food sensitivities. Although it has become commonplace to poke fun at people with such sensitivities, it is rarely either helpful or supportive.

CHAPTER 6

Bite on This

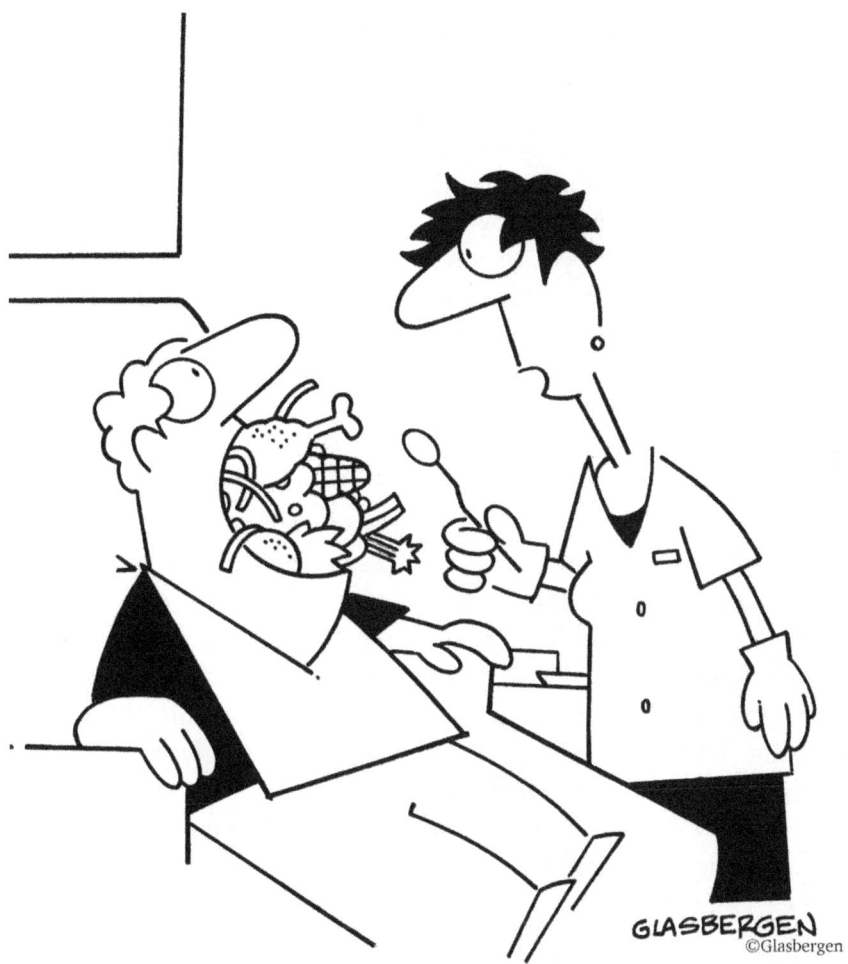

"You need to floss better."

O h, how much we loathe going to the dentist! The drills! The pain! The cost! The guilt! All that lying through your crumbling teeth! That you brush *at least* twice daily. Carry an interdental pikster in your wallet wherever you go. Floss like a demon every morning and night. It's true, Your Worship, you garble upon all that is holy – while your dentist prods about in the holey-mess of your uncherished biters and sighs over your galloping gum recession.

What's a dentist to do? They know that you know that they know you're winging it. Bent on spinning your lousy dental care into myth to avoid what you hear as *the lecture* and what the dentist delivers as *professional instruction to enhance the longevity of your dentition*. It's a thin line a dentist treads. As it is for any health professional who's dedicated years of study to helping and improving people who just will not be helped or improved. Just like you, they have rent, mortgages, school fees and a lifestyle to fund. But, unlike you, if it all goes wrong, and you leave your entire set of teeth embedded in an apple or swallow a few of them down with a piece of steak, *they* can't sue *you* for your own negligence!

You'll notice that so far, I've avoided using the L-word in regard to how we relate to our dentists (L being short for *lying*... dictionary definition, '*not telling the truth*'). I'm not even sure dentists use it themselves, actually. No matter how dispassionate their professional eye. No matter how many times they fruitlessly repeat the mantra – 'Let's fix the *small* problems before they become *big* problems, shall we?' Or what surprise bits of meals-long-past they discover wedged under your swollen gum-line. How abundant the plaque. How eye-watering the state of your breath. How frustratingly fixable these problems can be and, in truth, *are*. Because the main consolation as your dentist's Porsche purrs into their palatial homestead's parking bay after a hard day slaving over hot mouths is that they *depend* upon your casual, unthinking neglect.

And before you start twisting this inability to call you out for that neglect into a case for co-dependence and enabling, I personally consider it a survival skill, common to most health professionals. Let's just say, I have yet to meet a dentist, faced with a well-cared for mouth, who *wouldn't* be the first to exclaim in sheer wonderment, 'Oh, what a marvellous example of the glorious benefits of daily dental care!'. Like, if they ever saw one.

It's quite a thrill to be told by a dentist or periodontist that your gums are the best they've seen in a while, let me tell you. I know this firsthand because it happened to me only a few months ago. I'd totally reversed my smallish but potentially catastrophic inflamed gum problem with a rotating head electric toothbrush over a few months. Well, that and upgrading my flossing to twice a day! The poor man seemed genuinely touched that someone had so minutely followed his instructions and solved their own problem. We were both, albeit briefly, bathed in the glow of virtue. A win/win situation all around.

Perhaps this was partly because more than 90% of Australian adults delay scheduling a dental check-up until that small quick-fixable problem has escalated into a monster. Until the pain of toothache, decay and gum disease is unbearable. And, even then, most people delay the visit. Despite gum disease being known as the biggest cause of tooth loss. In fact, some people delay until they're hospitalised with tooth abscesses and blood poisoning. All of which suggests that, in our efforts to save money, time and discomfort, we're monumentally failing to notice how much our dental procrastination is actually costing us. Like 'shutting the stable door after the horse has bolted' – as my Grandmother would have said.

A Noah's Ark dental joke goes like this:

> *Patient: 'Must I really floss my teeth, doctor?'*
> *Dentist: 'Only the ones you want to keep...'*

So, given that the most basic benefits of dental health are fresher breath, painless chewing, prevention of tooth and gum loss, as well as cleaner, whiter, more attractive teeth, why do you suppose – in this pouting, selfie-taking age – the concept of daily dental discipline is so low on the average person's grooming and self-care radar? Especially, when you consider that we already have reams of research detailing gum disease as a primary precursor to heart disease, stroke, dementia and diabetes? Furthermore, if you're thinking of just having them all ripped out eventually and replaced with a denture – or you can afford a mouth full of implants – what happens when your dental care has been so poor your gums and jawbone won't form a solid base for either dentures or implants?

Strangely, and not so very long ago, preventive dentistry did actually call for having all your teeth removed to prevent tooth problems. Terrifying as it may sound now, it was a common strategy. In fact, less than 100 years ago, in my Grandmother's day that's precisely what she did. Unfortunately, neither she nor her dentist factored in the shock to her body of removing her entire mouth's complement of perfectly healthy teeth. Especially, as there were no dental anaesthetics in those days except laudanum. The lack of both antibiotic cover and formal oral hygiene training of the day further compounded her discomfort. Her gums became inflamed and infected and she was sick as a dog for months. Reduced to soft foods like bread soaked in milk because she couldn't chew at all, her general health began to suffer. Her previously healthy gums shrank and when she did finally get her promised 'new teeth' they didn't fit so well and soon became loose, making chewing even more tricky. Nor was she given any instruction on caring for her dentures other than soaking them in salty water. And, at the time, it was assumed that without teeth there was no need to brush anything in the mouth to keep it clean. My Grandmother had trouble with her dentures until the day she died and always regretted following the advice of her so-called *modern* dentist of the 1920s.

For the past 40 years at least, dentists have focused on preventive dentistry, gum disease and restorative work. Old-fashioned mercury laden amalgam fillings have all but disappeared, replaced by tooth coloured composite fillings which are less toxic and more natural to look at. In the 1980s forward thinking dentists began to employ hygienists to further educate their clients in basic dental care and how to keep your teeth for as long as possible. The arrival of the digital age in the 1990s, however, appears to have undone much progress in common sense health care across the board – encouraging a belief in instant fixes and cosmetic replacements in a modern version of my Grandmother's experience in the 1920s. But despite all the miracle innovations and information available since the 1990s, we are still not brushing our teeth with anything like the frequency required to keep them.

When I hear one of my clients say something like – 'I don't have time to brush my teeth… let alone floss every day' – I know they've seriously lost the plot. Since when is anyone too busy to spend one or two minutes brushing their teeth? Unless you're under heavy artillery fire and trapped in a bunker, my answer to clients who are too busy to brush their teeth usually runs something like this… 'Well, you'll soon be needing to make time to puree your food then.' Funny how we can make time to surf the net, post cute cat memes on social media, sink a beer or a cocktail though. None of which will be of much comfort when we can't chew. Okay, maybe the cat memes.

Then there's this – 'I've always had a naughty sweet tooth. Especially at night. I love the taste of chocolate as I fall asleep.' Quite aside from the choking hazard of falling asleep with lumps of chocolate melting in your mouth, there's the ghastly damage that occurs when you leave sugar in a sleeping mouth without the usual cleansing rinse of saliva. Because, you see, your salivary glands need to 'sleep' too. Not totally, maybe. But enough to fail to dilute and rinse away the acids and sugars slowly dissolving your tooth enamel and inflaming your gums.

Georgie was one of those people who loved falling asleep with a sweet in her mouth. She also loved red wine and coffee. And her idea of cleaning her teeth was to bypass brushing altogether and go for the convenience of a quick rinse with a pretty heavy-duty mouth wash upon rising. Needless to say, she suffered inflamed gums and had endured extensive dental work most of her life. Her teeth were also very discoloured. When a diagnosis of bipolar disorder finally galvanised her into taking better care of herself it was the proverbial blessing in disguise. While we worked on improving her nutrition and gradually eliminating the mood altering, tooth-dissolving sugar from her diet, I offset at least some of her resistance with a quick fix of sorts. Of a dental sort, really. Something she'd be able to see in a couple of weeks which would cheer her up and give her a tangible health benefit. I got her flossing and brushing with a rotating head electric toothbrush topped with one of the best whitening toothpastes around. The combination of gum massage, plaque and food debris removal and whitening was dramatic. Two weeks later, as promised, her teeth and gums were truly transformed. Not perfect, I might add. But transformed enough to make her want to continue.

As you can probably tell, I'm a big fan of rotating head electric toothbrushes. I didn't used to be. Frankly, and I'm ashamed to say it, I thought electric toothbrushes were for wankers. You know the sort. People who have a gadget for everything – like digital carving knives and can openers and mobile phone apps to remind them to have a drink of water every now and then.

I'm also a big fan of dental tape, rather than the thinner floss. This is because the tape seems gentler on gums which are not yet used to daily flossing. Don't be alarmed if your gums bleed a little first time around either. That's normal if they're unused to being flossed. In no time at all your gums will toughen up and stop bleeding.

Like most dentists, I'm not a big fan of harsh mouthwashes. Many of them contain alcohol which strips the mouth somewhat of its protective coating of slipperiness. In any case, mouthwashes are no replacement for twice daily brushing.

While we're on the subject of brushing, ask your dentist or their hygienist to show you how to brush the crud off your teeth professionally. It won't take long and can save you a lot of grief down the track. Most of us were simply handed a toothbrush with some toothpaste on it as kids and told to get on with it. Consequently, most people are completely untrained in effective brush technique. So, corralling your dentist for some lessons will pay off handsomely in the long run.

Last of all, please make friends with your dentist. Remember that the better you look after your teeth the less traumatic your relationship will be.

CHAPTER 7

You Gotta Have Skin

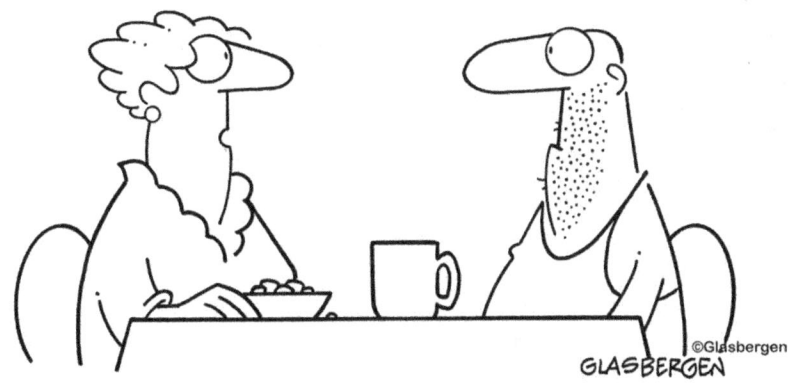

"Every day my body sheds millions of old skin cells and replaces them with fresh new cells. And you never even notice!

The day I sat down to write this chapter, I saw a news article about a baby boy born without skin on most of his tiny body. He had skin on only his head and parts of his legs. The skin on his neck, chest, back, arms, hands and feet was missing. At four months, the poor little mite had been in hospital for his entire life.

> 'The skin is our largest organ and has many important functions, such as protecting us from infection and keeping body temperature regulated,' a consulting dermatologist observed. 'When you don't have a good barrier, especially as a baby, you can run into a lot of different problems.'

A paediatric dermatologist commented, *'This child is going to have a very challenging life ahead of him'*.

'Even if he does pull through, we don't know what the future holds,' said the baby's mother. *'We're just praying every day. Every day is a blessing.'*

It's hard to imagine how we'd cope without the protective, waterproof, self-repairing, stretchable, temperature regulating, washable outer wrapping that covers almost every square millimetre of us. It's even more difficult to fathom where we might put several other vitally important parts of ourselves without it – like our hair, nails, pores, sweat and sebaceous glands, sensory nerves, various openings, etcetera. The vast majority of us have never known life without our miracle skin wrap and, unless something goes badly wrong with it, most people take it for granted.

Even if you do believe skin care is a vital element of your self-care routine, you'd be forgiven for thinking the only area of your skin that really matters is the skin from your neck upwards. Because most of the skin care information you see online or on TV or in magazines focuses solely on saving either your face or the front of your neck, right? You'd also be forgiven for thinking that lines, wrinkles, crepiness and any kind of dullness, puffiness or bumpiness are clear evidence of your abject failure to use the advertised products to cleanse, tone and moisturise. Which is all well and good until you realise those kinds of beliefs are untrue *and* leave the other 90% of your skin up the proverbial creek in terms of any kind of proper daily care. And that's only your outside skin. What about the kilometres of epithelium on your insides? The stuff that covers your bones and organs and other bits?

It may come as a surprise but the contents of each chapter of this book will help you do something which has the potential to improve *all* of your skin. Yes, 100%, all of it. However, strange as it might seem, many people who fork out a fortune for anti-ageing creams and rejuvenating treatments mostly don't bother too much about the natural everyday ways they can improve their skin all over because they're hooked on the mythical miracle quick-fix. Stranger still, although there's plenty of evidence that inexpensive skin care regimes work extremely well, many folks are either disbelieving or completely flummoxed by the utter simplicity of them.

With the global cosmetics market predicted to reach upwards of US$700 billion in 2024 – and the cosmetic surgery industry projected to reach at least US$44 billion by 2025 – we're not destined to be free of either beauty industry influence or its influencers anytime soon. So, don't get me started on the supposed supernatural benefits of those anti-ageing products and services touched by the magic wand of celebrity endorsement.

Be that as it may, it's when you compare the above figures to the mere US$332 billion invested in wind and solar energy in 2018 (down 8% from 2017!) that you get a glimpse of what humans (aka, *homo sapiens*, or 'wise man') regard as important these days. Good work, beauty industry marketing people. At least some of us will look hyper-real and Insta-ready as our planet goes to hell in a handbasket.

> 'Publishers don't generally sell magazines by reminding readers that nothing works. Consequently, getting straight answers about anti-ageing and beauty products is nearly impossible. There exists a confluence of fact-twisting forces: lots of money to be made by manufacturers and providers, huge advertising campaigns that deploy vast quantities of pseudoscientific gobbledygook, a lack of independent research and information, and consumers who desperately want the products to do for them what is claimed. The cumulative impact of all these forces results in a massive bias toward representing a product or procedure as effective. I call this the "beauty-industry efficacy bias," or BIEB for short.'
>
> **An adapted quote (published by *The Atlantic*) from *Is Gwyneth Paltrow Wrong About Everything?* by Timothy Caulfield – health, law & policy professor at the University of Alberta**

In any case, all the hyperbolic promises, celebrity endorsements, weird pseudoscientific ingredients and hope-in-a-jar that the beauty industry very profitably cooks up is nothing if not upwardly mobile. And the more competitive the market becomes, the more pressure on you to try, buy and apply. Never mind the old adage 'just because you can, doesn't mean you should' – it's well known that hardly anyone reads the 'terms and conditions', side-effects or contraindications anymore. Even the skin people, for the most part!

Interestingly, not once have I ever been asked by a dermatologist about my diet, exercise, hydration or sleep habits. Not once have I been asked if I smoke, use illicit drugs, scoff junk food daily or drink buckets of alcohol. Neither have I been asked these questions by any beauty therapist. Despite the usual protracted sigh over my 'sun damage', no dermatologist has recommended or offered me a sample of what they consider the ultimate non-greasy 50+ SPF sunscreen either. Although I can't say that any of them (with only *two* dermatologist exceptions) have been at all shy about recommending a raft of treatment plans and products which involve a tidy profit margin for themselves. The dermatology exceptions simply sent me back to the real world with an understanding that I'd got what could be expected at my age, a 'don't pick at the frozen sunspot scabs' and a 'see you in 12 months'. Given I began noticing this particular attitude when I was around 35 and still sporting the luminosity of skin that strangers complimented me upon in the street, I'd say disdain and profiteering are culturally entrenched in both the beauty and dermatology industries. And because women – and increasingly men – have been culturally conditioned to dread any signs of ageing, we are sitting ducks for the upsell.

So, while I encourage each and every person in Australia to have their skins thoroughly and regularly checked by a qualified dermatologist for basal cell carcinomas (BCCs), squamous cell carcinomas (SCCs), melanomas and anything else you're worried about – I urge you all to start asking yourself the very questions the skin boffins *are not* asking you. Because, whether you believe it or not, your skin is a brilliant outward reflection of how the rest of your precious body is muddling along under your care.

For example:

- How is your digestive health going? (pimples, acne, blackheads, rosacea, rashes)

- What is your liver up to? (acne, itchy skin, dull skin, yellowish tinge, redness, rashes)

- Does your thyroid need some help? (dry skin, hair loss, cold hands, flaky nails, vitiligo)

- If and where does your immune system need a boost? (hives, slow healing, infections, herpes, shingles, allergies)

- Does your insomnia need to be addressed? (lines, puffiness, dark eye circles, allergies, worsening eczema/psoriasis/acne, washed out complexion)

- What are your hormones up to? (acne, dryness, oiliness, milia, clogged hair follicles, inflammation)

All these things, and more, can be warning signs that you need to start paying attention to what's happening on your insides so you can start changing a few things to improve your outsides. Even if your genetic beauty inheritance is enough to make your favourite glamorous film star want to put a bag over their head! Even if, appearance-wise at least, you are currently getting away with burning your candles at both ends. Because, scarily, after 30, all that candlewax will come home to roost on your skin – if you'll forgive the mixed metaphor. And what for the less beautiful of us? Do what the French do. Look after yourself. Do the best with what you have. Vitality, a sense of humour, a fully functioning brain and a good night's sleep can do wonders for the getting of both attention and a glowing complexion. Don't leave home without them.

So how can you sort the help from the hype? Well, why not start here? With at least *some* of the input your skin needs to be the best you can make it without the chunky price tag. At least I'm not trying to flog you something you don't need. I'm just passing on a few commonsense skin care facts and tips, as I see them. In any case, wouldn't you like to know what to use on your skin if suddenly, for whatever reason, you could neither afford nor find all those commercial pots of so-called 'miracle' cream? Here's a hint. Most of it is – or should be – in your kitchen.

The following ideas won't cost you much, but they'll certainly improve the texture, colour and overall health of your skin – from tip to toe – in just four weeks.

12 daily skincare habits which will improve your skin in four weeks:

- ditch all junk food and drinks

- eat a fresh diet rich in colourful vegetables and fruits, light proteins, cold pressed oils, fermented foods

- snack on nuts, seeds and beansprouts

- drink water to hydrate your body and quench your thirst

- reduce or eliminate alcohol

- cleanse your face before you go to sleep

- *gently* exfoliate all over – use a dry natural bristle brush or shower with an exfoliating glove

- moisturise *all* over

- cover up in the hottest, brightest part of the day and use a 50+ sunscreen

- do some sort of exercise daily

- make time to relax

- get a good night's sleep.

10 skin treatments made from stuff you can find in your fridge or pantry:

- lactic acid face mask or bathwater softener – paint on plain probiotic yoghurt

- fruit acid face mask or body exfoliator – pawpaw juice painted on skin

- zit buster face mask – strawberry juice, plain probiotic yoghurt, pawpaw juice (one at a time or all at once)

- clarifying mask for face, neck and décolletage – organic honey and a few drops of lemon juice

- soothing facial spray – chilled rosewater

- avocado oil night treatment – massage into face and neck, or a dessert spoonful in a warm bath

- oatmeal exfoliator – blitz oats in food processor, soften with a little warm water or milk, apply with gentle, circular movements, rinse off

- soothing oatmeal bath – one cup of oatmeal in a muslin bag in warm bath

- cucumber cooling mask – use slices of cucumber or juice

- rice bran oil skin polisher – apply sparingly to damp, freshly exfoliated skin from face to feet.

A selection of foods that improve your skin:

- antioxidant berries – blueberries, strawberries, raspberries, blackberries, gooseberries, goji berries, cranberries

- yellow fruits – pawpaw, papaya, mango

- fruits with pectin – apples, pears, guavas, quince, citrus, cherries, grapes, strawberries

- yellow vegetables – carrots, pumpkin, sweet potato

- red vegetables – bell peppers, beetroot, tomatoes

- green vegetables – dark leafy greens, broccoli, French beans, kale, cabbage, spinach, celery, avocado

- fermented vegetables – sauerkraut and kimchi

- fermented dairy – yoghurt, lassi, buttermilk

- sustainable fish – especially oily fish, salmon, tuna, mackerel, herring, anchovies, pilchards, sardines

- nuts and seeds – walnuts, brazil nuts, almond, pumpkin seeds, sesame seeds, pepitas

- probiotics and prebiotic foods (see above and Chapter 3)

- whole grains, beans, legumes, cacao, miso.

FAQs

Why is my face so puffy and dull looking?

I hear this question a lot. But it's the wrong question. It's not the why, it's the what. As in, *'What* is making my face so puffy and dull looking?' Once you've sussed out the trigger or cause, the next logical question is *'When* will I stop doing it and look after myself better?'

Unless you're pregnant, unresolved celiac, doing IVF, on a course of corticosteroids, radiation, chemotherapy or immune suppressants, have kidney, liver or heart failure – facial puffiness, pastiness and/or fluid retention all over are usually related to excess consumption of sugary treats, salty treats, starchy treats, alcoholic treats and all the chemical additives, colourants and preservatives therein. Pointing this out to people is fraught with danger though – which is probably why most therapists (including doctors) don't go there. Neither does it matter if people are paying you actual money to tell them the truth, the whole truth and nothing but. They don't want to know that it's their gut microbiome crying out for a break and some pre and probiotics. They don't want to hear this even when the indications are right there in their aching joints, headaches and the pages of their food diaries, as well as their skin. It's easier to just stop keeping a food diary and pretend that devilish triumvirate of puffiness, dullness and fluid retention are simply unfair, random afflictions, fixable by something other than sheer willpower and an avoidance of deliciously addictive triggers. Sorry, but you *did* ask.

Should I start injectables like Botox and fillers early so I can just 'zap' the lines and wrinkles before they come?

It depends what you mean by 'early'. But why would anyone be spending their hard-earned on 'zapping' wrinkles you can't even see yet? In my opinion, much of what can be *effectively* achieved with muscle freezing, fillers, lasers, skin peels and more invasive cosmetic surgery, needs to be put through at least *one* of the following filters and, in truth, probably *all* of them:

- Are you under the age of 35?

- Do you have a genuinely disfiguring skin condition which could truly benefit from some well-administered and subtle professional help?

- Does your lifestyle support your general health?

- Are you expecting a quick cosmetic fix for self-inflicted skin damage which you've enthusiastically acquired over and above what might be considered normal wear and tear?

- Are you trying to achieve the photoshopped perfection of celebrities and models in beauty and fashion magazines?

- Have you researched who is doing the work, their qualifications and what products they're really using?

What's wrong with wanting to look like someone famous, if you can afford to get some 'work' done?

Beneath all the filters and styling tricks employed to elevate the glamour pusses of TV-streaming-world to the realms of the super-rich, it's entirely possible that they are perfectly nice people with barely a zit, wrinkle or centimetre of cellulite between them. Howsoever, when the *swodge* of fads for which I hold them almost singlehandedly responsible starts teenagers (or 20-somethings) prematurely fretting about non-existent crow's-feet, thus propelling them into clinics for Botox, fillers, butt 'n' breast enhancements and permanent eyebrow tattooing? Surely, someone's got to draw a line somewhere before we *all* become Kardashian clonebots with identical enhanced pouts, arched black brows, cinched waists and fake lashes worn during daylight hours? Because it seems to me that we've now reached *#PeakBeautyIndustryBullShit*! The sort of *#industrialstrengthBS* that promises much but delivers so very little of deep importance. Even the invincible Kim Kardashian appears jack of it, having recently jumped the *#selfie-ship* and tottered off to law school! (Well, for a couple of weeks, anyway. Barely an Instagram nanosecond elapsed before she'd appeared at the Met Gala with an impossibly tiny waist, launched her new shapewear range and insulted the Japanese by appropriating a cultural icon for the brand name.)

So cosmetic injectables are bad?

Firstly, the muscle paralysing effect of Botox and products like it can also be highly effective for a variety of medical conditions – chronic migraines, Bell's palsy, thyroid eye disease, excessive sweating, hyper-salivation, spasmodic dysphonia (a neurological condition affecting the vocal cords), crossed eyes and eyelid spasms. So, I'm not saying that using fillers and Botox (including similar *botulinum toxin* products like Dysport, Myobloc and Xeomin) is all bad. Just that teenagers and 20-somethings are self-conscious enough without the beauty industry telling them they *need* cosmetic injectables. Sparingly applied, genuine cosmetic injectables can and do boost both appearance and confidence – but can we not just save these treatments for grown-ups? You know, the people who don't necessarily fancy showcasing a lifetime of stress, sleeplessness and erstwhile habits indelibly etched into their 50-year-old faces, making them look closer to 70. Fifty being the new 30, you understand.

Nevertheless, there's a tendency to freeze 'n' fill 'n' tighten 'n' laser resurface *everything* these days which is resulting in even older people all looking the same. The evidence is all around you. Those frozen faces, immovable eyebrows, tight-slightly-boiled-looking cheeks and puffy pouts don't come naturally to *anyone* between 40 and 75. Less is certainly more – but restraint and subtlety seem in short supply when there's a sale to be made.

Do I really need to exfoliate?

In my opinion, if you really want to keep your skin in tip-top condition, exfoliation is a must. Every day you lose millions of dead skin cells. In fact, the very top layer of your epidermis – the *stratum corneum* – is made up of dead skin cells. These cells have worked their way to the surface to be sloughed off by your clothes, items you touch and that touch you, through movement and washing. This sloughing off of skin cells throughout the day is *natural* exfoliation. But if you want to help the process and have your moisturisers work better for you, try gently exfoliating your skin, showering off the debris and then applying your moisturiser to a slightly damp skin. You'll find your moisturiser works better and for longer. You'll find less 'skin dust' in your house and on your clothes. Exfoliation also helps prevent milia[5] and blocked pores, as well as stimulating blood circulation to your skin. The trick is to exfoliate gently several times a week as part of your normal showering routine. You don't need fancy scrubs. All you need is a soft bristle brush or an exfoliating glove. And a word of warning – please don't attack your skin like a bull at a gate. You'll just cause a lot of unnecessary redness and probably even some damage.

Let's take a look at a couple of my clients who reaped the benefits of my practice of simple skin care from the inside out and the divine aromatherapy facial…

Sandra came to see me to help clarify her skin eight weeks before her wedding. She was concerned about dark circles under her eyes, the scattering of milia across her cheeks, as well as angry spots on her back and chin which she couldn't resist picking at. Because I knew she worked long, unsociable hours as a theatre nurse in a large city hospital I asked her to keep a food and fluids diary for 10 days before her appointment. Despite her protests that she already ate a fresh healthy diet and 'not much' junk or sugar, I insisted.

'Oh, no,' she groaned. 'Then you'll be able to see what I'm eating.'

'Precisely the point,' I replied, laughing. But because she had the build of a small bird and losing weight for the big day was unnecessary, I added, 'It's just to see if we need to add anything to help your skin look fresher. The good news is you don't have to worry about amounts… unless you devour an entire block of chocolate, bowl of chips or packet of Tim Tams in one sitting.'

---

[5] Milia are small, yellow or white cysts about 1-2mm in size found under the skin. They usually appear in clusters, mostly commonly on the face around the eyelids and cheeks. They can also appear on the back and shoulders. Milia are often found in newborns but can affect people of any age.

As it turned out, Sandra's food diary was a revelation. Sugary snacks had snuck into her routine a minimum of three times a day. It appeared the only regular fresh vegetable matter she consumed, other than a bit of salad on a sandwich, was when visiting her mother on Sundays. Aside from frequent cups of coffee, her fluid intake was appallingly small. She was also persistently constipated. Like many theatre nurses she was chronically dehydrated, living on adrenaline and bolstering her energy with quick fixes of sugar and coffee.

- We began with my 21 Foods a Day routine. I detailed how she could throw seven fresh food items into a bowl or a hot pan three times a day to achieve it.

- I suggested she take a probiotic at night to help rebalance her digestive tract.

- To help with chronic dehydration, constipation and the dark circles under her eyes, I suggested she start drinking 250ml (one teacup) of fresh water every hour in the spaces between going into theatre and especially directly afterwards when she was done for the day.

- We then moved onto applying clarifying aromatherapy facials and back treatments once a week for the first month. The facials consisted of exfoliation, milia removal, resolution of whiteheads and white clay masks with a balancing blend of essential oils of lavender and rose geranium to suit her hypersensitive skin. Anti-inflammatory massage and gentle lymphatic drainage massage, especially around the eyes, was also included.

- Whiteheads on her back were removed and a white clay mask with a blend of lavender, frankincense and rose geranium was applied to her back for 30 minutes before being washed off and spritzed with rosewater. She was instructed to use a dry natural bristle brush on her back twice a week before showering.

Four weeks later, Sandra told me she felt like a changed woman. She was planning her meals ahead and her nutrition was vastly improved. What's more, she was enjoying her food and her energy levels were better without the blood sugar spikes of sugary treats. She was convinced the elimination of sugary treats and the hydration was helping her feel less anxious about the wedding preparations too. She was particularly thrilled that the spots and marks on her back were resolving because she'd chosen an almost entirely backless dress for her wedding gown. With the exception of a brief sugary hiccup during her hen's celebrations, Sandra stayed on the straight and narrow for a second month. On her wedding day, she was free to love every minute of the ceremony, reception and close-up photography without worrying about having to hide her skin. In a video posted online, she looked radiant.

Noreen originally came to see me for a simple lash and brow tint. She was 55, well dressed and groomed. The first thing I noticed about her was a cast on her right arm. The second was an outbreak of what looked like rosacea around her nostrils and across her cheeks. As I tinted her brows and lashes, her story unfolded. She was having her brows and lashes dyed because she could no longer apply her make-up with her right hand. The arm had been badly broken when she'd slipped on a spill in a corridor at work, resulting in significant nerve, tendon and skin damage. Despite multiple surgeries over 18 months, the insertion of a plate and even a skin graft, her arm was still not right. She'd also suffered a staph infection beneath the plate in her arm and had been on many repeats of heavy-duty antibiotics for 15 months. To top it off, she was looking at several more surgeries and the possibility of even more antibiotics in the coming years.

When I asked her about the red rash across her nose and cheeks, she told me her GP had diagnosed rosacea and given her a script for antibiotics. She'd tried but couldn't take them, she said, because they made her feel sick. So, I told her that I was also a trained beauty therapist, specialising in natural skin care and asked her if she'd give me a chance to help her resolve the rash.

- We started with an overhaul of her nutrition to the 21 Foods a Day plan which should include as much yoghurt, berries and fresh vegetables as possible.

- I recommended a course of probiotics to be taken at night so the good bacteria could work their magic on her gut microbiome overnight.

- I also suggested she start eating a slice of ripe pawpaw every morning before anything else and that she should paint some of the juice on her face while she was doing it. An unusual request, but I've found that an enzyme in pawpaw called 'papain' is very good for clearing both the digestive system and the surface of the epidermis. I call it the 'garbage eating enzyme' because, essentially, that's what it does.

- She then booked in for an aromatherapy facial in which I used essential oils such as German chamomile and frankincense – mixed into an anti-inflammatory massage oil, hydrosols, gels and my favourite gentle white clay mask – to soothe away the redness and inflammation on the outside just as her new pro and prebiotic rich diet was doing on her insides.

- For use in between sessions, I made her a bespoke aromatherapy range of relatively inexpensive skin care. An anti-inflammatory cleanser, a rose and lavender hydrosol spritz and a soothing rebalancing gel that I'd originally formulated from aloe vera gel and essential oils for long haul flights and jet lag.

It took a few months to get Noreen's digestive system back on track after all the antibiotics she'd had but, combined with her new daily skin care routine and her monthly facials, her skin was finally completely free of the nasty red rash. And remains so to this day.

CHAPTER 8

Float Like a Butterfly: Surprising Links Between Posture, Balance & Strength

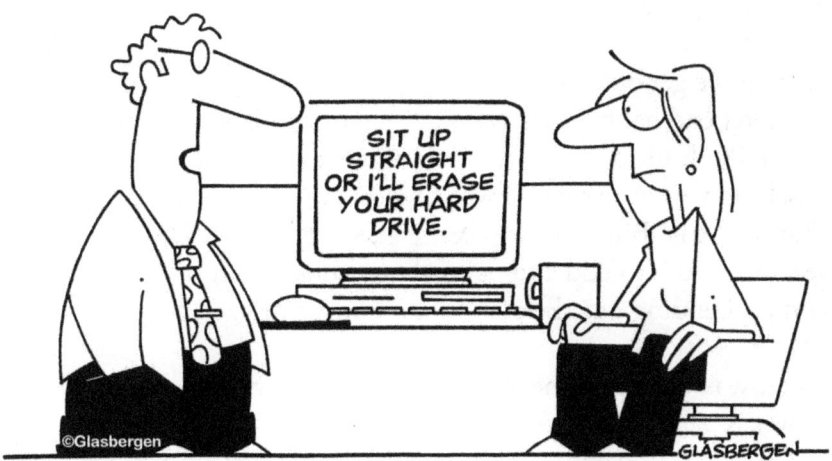

"It's called Ergonomics."

For thousands of years it's been no secret that a person's posture both influences and showcases their self-perception. Imagine how far Marcus Aurelius might have got if he'd been seen slumping through the Roman Senate. Or if a single Roman-oppressed Celt would have bothered following the legendary Boadicea into battle if she'd been flopped on a couch while detailing her revolutionary battle technique of attaching sharp knives at knee height to her war chariots. In fact, so charismatic was Boadicea – Queen of the Iceni – that ancient sources recorded tribes who wouldn't normally have supported an Iceni-led attack plan jumped at the chance of joining her revolt against the Romans. I'd like to think her posture and bearing had something to do with that.

It's also well known among singers, actors, politicians and most people in the public eye that good posture not only commands the respect of your audience but also reduces aches and pains, decreases stress, prevents repetitive injury and even improves your mood. So why is it that the average person mostly thinks of posture in terms of their mother nagging them to, 'for god sakes, dear, stand up straight – you look like a pudding'?

Later, as we get older and there's no-one who cares enough to nag us anymore, bad habits such as slouching and collapsing in front of the TV or PC lead to awkward walking styles, and weak and fatigued muscles as well. And every time we repeat our poor posture habits, guess what happens? Bingo! Our posture gets even worse. Until eventually we're hogtied into odd and painful positions by our own muscles and tendons bending our skeleton into a human pretzel.

When was the last time you thought about your posture? If your answer is *never*, you're certainly not alone.

Take the time to look around you when you're out and about and you'll see plenty of examples of people who've never given their posture a moment's thought. Hunched shoulders. Forward heads. Bowed upper backs. Swayed lower backs. Slumped spines. Awkward side-to-side gaits. Ask pretty much anyone with poor posture how they're feeling, and you'll find they're almost always in some sort of pain or discomfort. Their largely unconscious adapted ways of standing, sitting and carrying themselves almost always accompanied by one or more side-effects caused by the compensations that poor posture forces you to adopt just so you can get about.

Compensations that just creep up on you while you're busy doing something else. Side effects you've probably never even considered were connected to your increasingly uncomfortable choice to lug your precious body around like a sack of spuds. Like waddling, continually scuffing or shuffling your feet, frequent trips, falls and skids. Or shallow breathing, leg weakness, lower back ache, 'texting neck', sore shoulders. Maybe a stabbing sciatic nerve, knee and hip joint pain, dodgy ankles and plantar fasciitis. And on top of all that the gradual worsening of old injuries, headaches, migraines, aggravation of tinnitus and those debilitating twinges in your hands, wrists or arms that mimic carpal tunnel syndrome.

And that's not the end of it. Poor posture causes changes in how your muscles work together. Shortening some muscles, lengthening others to gradually pull your skeleton clean off its natural centre. This causes problems with your balance that, when combined with inactivity, can throw you quite literally *right off balance*. But having good balance is really important for your health, not just because you're less like to fall over but also because it keeps your nerve pathways and muscles functioning in the coordinated way they should. So good balance and posture also help keep your muscles strong.

> 'Our balance declines as we age because our muscles become weaker and the inner-ear receptors that sense movement stiffen. But everybody can get better with practice.'
> **Daniel Ferris, PhD,**
> **professor of movement science &**
> **director of Human Neuromechanics Laboratory**
> **at the University of Michigan, USA**

Poor posture doesn't only wear out your body faster than normal ageing by forcing inappropriate weight loads through your joints – it messes with your mind too. Because poor posture interferes with your breathing, energy levels and general wellbeing by depriving you of your full requirement of oxygen. It also flattens your vital life force. Or, as Oriental medicine calls it your chi, ki or qi.

All that said, poor posture isn't necessarily *only* caused by unconscious and lax habits – even though it's almost always *maintained* by them. Tension, trauma, injury, stress, anxiety, depression, six weeks in a moon boot after a leg fracture, walking on crutches, post-operative immobilisation of any sort, etcetera, can all play a part in altering your posture. Essentially, if your posture was great before a debilitating event, you have a good chance of retrieving it by turning on your old nerve pathways with specific exercises when you're working towards being well again. This is one of the reasons why the new wave of orthopaedic surgeons insist on *pre*-hab training prior to knee and hip surgery, as well as post-operative rehabilitation. And it's one of the many reasons athletes, sportspeople and dancers seem to heal faster than couch potatoes. However, if your posture was shot before the unfortunate event, you'll have to learn the strengthening basics of good posture from scratch.

As with most things we learn in life, we all have to start from where we are. Although, on the plus side, the less you know, the more it is possible to learn. Perhaps the reason why people show such small interest in their posture is because it's what I like to call 'a foundation skill'. Not quite as vital for your body as breathing but at least as important as walking, listening and being able to sniff out what's good or poisonous for you. To our great detriment, many of us have already lost many of our foundation skills through taking them for granted, unhelpful lifestyle habits and, nowadays, encroaching automation. We've come to believe we don't need to attend to the basics our bodies are crying out for us to fix with good old *analog* attention. Nevertheless, whether you are fully functional, young, elderly, injured or disabled, learning how to manage your posture around your daily requirements and activities is vitally important to keep you looking youthful, strong, maintain your balance, reduce pain, and mitigate wear and tear.

Managing your posture will help you maintain correct form while exercising, resulting in fewer injuries and better results as you use the correct muscles for the job, rather than knee-jerking through your routine using inappropriate and unconscious compensatory techniques. Managing your posture by learning a few simple exercises will improve your balance, help prevent falls *and* improve your abilities in tennis, golf, running, dancing, skiing, climbing and a zillion other activities we upright homo sapiens like to do. Managing your posture will also boost your confidence, clear your head and lift your mood by simply allowing your life force to flow more freely – as opposed to being scrunched up, lopsided and intermittent.

Essentially there are three key areas to focus on to successfully alter your posture:

- *Become aware* of postural problems – usually precipitated by injury or necessity

- *Learn how to fine tune* everyday movements and stances – for example, standing, sitting, walking, strength and flexibility exercises

- *Daily practice and integration* – slow corrective movements consciously integrated into everyday movements to increase coordination and balance, as well as to gently move the body out of pain.

'Nothing ever goes away until it teaches us what we need to know.'

**Pema Chödrön,
author, teacher & Buddhist Nun**

So, what *are* the basics of good posture? Standing up straight is a good start! However, as children many of us were told to *stand up rigidly straight and pull back our shoulders* in the military style. Fortunately, both cultural and therapeutic views on good posture have changed from those times, although many people still consider the military stance as the gold standard. It isn't, of course. When I see this sort of 'military' posture in my practice, it almost certainly comes with chronically contracted muscles in the shoulders, upper and lower back, buttocks and hamstrings. In addition, a raised chin tilts the head backwards, contracting the rear neck muscles. Consequently, many of them suffer regular nagging headaches, as well as chronic neck, jaw and back pain. I've also noticed that people who habitually stand like this are often perfectionists with a tendency towards anxiety. Their breathing might be quite shallow as they are rarely ever truly relaxed. They're also often quite resistant to the idea of standing up straight in a relaxed and balanced state because it just doesn't seem difficult or disciplined or perfect enough.

At the other end of the scale is the idea that good posture is 'hard work so why bother?' – this is as common as the notion that you can get by perfectly well without attending to your posture *at all*. I suppose if you're very young, perhaps you can. Just look at how marvellously well-balanced young children are. It's as if, once they get the hang of working with the forces of gravity – with what the physios call *neutral spine* and I call *the postural lightness of being* – they're unstoppable. How that lightness of being gradually begins to go to pot when the hormones kick in from around 12 or 13 is anyone's guess.

> 'Sitting is more dangerous than smoking, kills more people than HIV and is more treacherous than parachuting. We are sitting ourselves to death. The chair is out to kill us.'
>
> **James Levine,
> professor of medicine at the Mayo Clinic,
> in an interview with the *LA Times***

FAQs

I'm not sporty. And I'm not a fan of aerobics. What fun activities can I do for better posture, balance and strength?

Falling caused by loss of postural strength and balance is one of the biggest problems as we age. However, falling is also a growing problem for the young, distracted as they are while bent over mobile phones and tablets.

The following disciplines are a great start to retrieving your posture, balance and strength at almost any age. Each can be adapted to suit your age, lifestyle and ability. Each will challenge you in its own special way. The main techniques they all share are awareness, breathing, stretching, standing and improvement of your central core strength. Rediscovering your core strength can be a revelation. No matter how unfit or overweight you are. Or, conversely, how fit and fabulous you are.

Yoga – There are many forms of yoga so experiment until you find the class you enjoy. If you're a beginner start with a beginner's class to learn the basic forms. Yoga helps individuals of all ages reconnect to their body. Yoga also helps train the body into correct posture by showing you how to become more aware of your breathing and what your body is telling you. Yoga strengthens the body and teaches step-by-step processes to help individuals tolerate sensations as they stretch and learn various positions called *asanas*. It also encourages awareness of stresses and potential strains.

Tai Chi – Tai Chi forms, Shibashi and specialised Tai Chi Falls Prevention classes are functional, challenging and fun ways to improve your posture, core stability and balance, memory, awareness and strength. I particularly like the emphasis on maintaining balance and awareness while moving because most damaging problems occur while we are moving *without* awareness. Balancing on one leg, shifting weight from one side of your body to another, elegant turning techniques, stability while changing direction and the discovery of your own centre of gravity await you! After a few months you'll find yourself using Tai Chi moves in all sorts of everyday situations. One study found that a small group of practitioners in their late 60s scored over 90% on measures of stability after a period of Tai Chi practice. Other research has shown that regular practice can reduce falls by up to 45%. A word of warning though – Tai Chi may look excruciatingly slow but it's harder than it looks! In fact, the slower you practice it, the harder it is, the stronger you become.

Somatics – Somatic therapies and disciplines are sometimes called the 'Yogas of the West'. Somatic practices include Feldenkrais, Alexander technique, Body-Mind Centering, Ortho-Bionomy, Pilates, yoga and Tai Chi. Clinical Somatics, however, originally developed by Thomas

Hanna, is neuromuscular or nerve-muscle education designed to relieve chronic pain and prevent recurring injuries by re-educating the nervous system with gentle exercise and a stretching technique called *pandiculation* (watch carefully and you'll see that cats, dogs, lions and tigers *pandiculate* all the time). Google your area to find one-on-one classes and group classes.

Pilates – Pilates is a system of total body exercises developed almost 100 years ago by Joseph Pilates to rehabilitate injured World War 1 soldiers. It is still recognised as an excellent strength, posture and conditioning discipline for professional dancers and sportspeople. The traditional method is low impact with an emphasis on precision of technique, postural alignment, core strength and controlled flowing movements using the breath to centre the mind. Classes are available one-on-one (which I recommend for beginners) or in groups.

Tango – Or simply take up the tango! As with *all* variations of ballroom dancing, the Tango has it all! Posture, dynamic balance, strength, static poses, nerve pathway renewal, awareness, attitude, confidence, coordination – but with great shoes, exquisite outfits and wonderful music.

Now let's take a look at some practical examples of postural training from my practice.

I first saw Bronwyn when she came to me for massage and leg strengthening training after substantial melanoma surgery to her right thigh in the early 2000s. We'd worked for a few years on massaging away her lower back pain, then retraining and strengthening her injured thigh, which had a square hole of surgical excision of muscle measuring some 12cms square and 4cms deep - essentially decommissioning most of her quads on that side. Then, after her children started high school and she'd gone back to work full-time, I didn't see her again for several years until, out of the blue, she called. She sounded stressed.

'I've just been told I need major spinal surgery,' she told me. 'I'm a bit scared and I'm in a lot of pain. Can I come and see you?' I asked her to bring her X-rays, scans and reports. She was certainly in a lot of pain and had been for some months. But something about her forward bend posture and side-to-side gait as she walked in told me to investigate further. I asked her if she'd be willing to postpone the surgery for a few months so we could give a combination of remedial massage techniques, postural and gait retraining a try. When I told her that the remedial massage element would involve hot stones and analgesic essential oils at the end of every session, she was in.

The first postural session involved teaching Bronwyn how to stand in neutral spine to take the weight off her lumbar/sacral spine and, hopefully, begin to turn off the stabbing pain from her sciatic nerve. It also included some gentle standing exercises to reposition her sacroiliac joints which she could do every time she felt a twinge. The remedial massage session included a slow and easy iliopsoas (major hip flexor often involved in either slight or pronounced bent over posture) release technique that relieved the drag on her anterior lumbar spine. Magically, the pain in her back was gone. Although it returned several days later as her adaptive postural habits kicked back in.

The second session involved much the same routine but with the addition of wall squats to strengthen her thigh muscles on both sides. Wall squats are a classic leg strengthening exercise for skiers. They are also very useful for strengthening the thighs of people who are too injured or uncoordinated to do either wide leg squats or standard width squats. This time the massage session also included instruction on how to stretch every muscle insertion and attachment into the pelvis, hip and leg we could find, as well as the lower back muscle release executed by releasing her major hip flexor.

The third session involved classic Tai Chi falls prevention techniques such as - weight shifting and turning, balancing on one leg while lifting the other, and the graceful, exquisitely slow Tai Chi walking style, both forwards and backwards. It also involved instruction for entering and exiting her car, stretches to relieve muscular tightness while sitting at her computer in her job as an accountant, the rolling of shoulders to release the neck and upper back, and seated butt stretches. Followed again by a soothing remedial massage and hip flexor release.

As I write, it's now 18 months since Bronwyn came to see me. She's lost 15 kilos *and* her side-to-side gait. She does her prescribed stretching exercises daily. She's able to go walking for daily exercise. Best of all, her chronic back pain is gone. Surgery is no longer required to fix the problem.

Jeremy rang to ask if I could do anything for his horrible headaches. He was a man in his mid-50s and used state-of-the-art hearing aids to counteract his growing deafness. Jeremy was embarrassed about his hearing loss and didn't want anyone, outside of his family, to know about it – which flagged me to look for compensatory postures and muscle contractions. When he told me he also had the annoying condition of tinnitus (incessant ringing or buzzing in the ears) I was even more interested to see how his deafness was affecting his upper body posture. The first examination revealed how he craned his head forward and slightly sideways to hear with his better ear. It also revealed how he twisted his entire torso and craned his neck to turn his better ear to the person who was speaking. His shoulders, neck, jaw and temple were so tight with tension that it was no wonder Jeremy was suffering such horrible daily headaches.

We began our course of postural training and remedial massage sessions by teaching Jeremy how to stand in relaxed but engaged neutral spine. This was followed by TMJ (temporomandibular joint) release exercises, neck and trapezius release exercises, listening position exercises and postural instruction for all. Naturally, all these techniques were backed up by soothing and pleasurable remedial massage with analgesic essential oils such as German chamomile.

The results were interesting. As long as Jeremy was able to maintain a daily discipline of postural techniques and release exercises, he was headache free. Even his tinnitus diminished by around 40%! A wonderful result *but*... as soon as he reverted to the same habits which had brought him to me? POW! The symptoms returned. Jeremy remains a work in progress.

Enid is one of my best examples of how ballroom dancing can actually change lives.

Enid was referred to me by her GP for aromatherapy and lymphatic drainage massage to ease her severe depression and deal with the fluid retention in her legs. A year before she'd suffered a stroke and it had taken five days for someone to discover her, lying on the floor of her living room. She was 85. She was lucky to be alive at all.

For the first several months I did house calls to her home in a retirement village every week. The main work was lymphatic drainage to relieve the oedema in her lower legs caused by her blood pressure drugs… and trying to get her laughing again.

After a while, I learned she'd signed up with a ballroom dancing class in the city. The staff at the retirement village were aghast that a woman who'd suffered such an insult to her life expectancy had suddenly taken it upon herself to schlepp into town twice a week to go ballroom dancing. There was nothing they could do to stop her though. So, everyone just held their collective breath until she arrived back safely.

Eventually, she told me she no longer wished me to come to the retirement village for her lymphatic drainage and relaxation treatments. She was now ready to come to me.

The first day she came to my clinic, she was so entranced by my aquarium and the beautiful fish therein, she suddenly walked towards it before I could either warn her to watch the step down to the level or get to her to grab her by the arm. And then something quite marvellous happened. Instead of crashing face-first off the step and into the aquarium... Enid executed the perfect ballroom dancing foil. *She took the next step* and saved her own self. Just six short months of ballroom dancing had taught her that. At 85.

Turns out you *can* teach an old brain new tricks. But if you want to invest in your future... why not start now? In my experience older people – from the 50s to even the over 80s – regain muscle strength at an astonishing rate if they put their mind to it. Often, it's simply a matter of encouragement and finding the right teacher. Same as the rest of us. So never say you're too old.

CHAPTER 9

Move It… or Lose It!

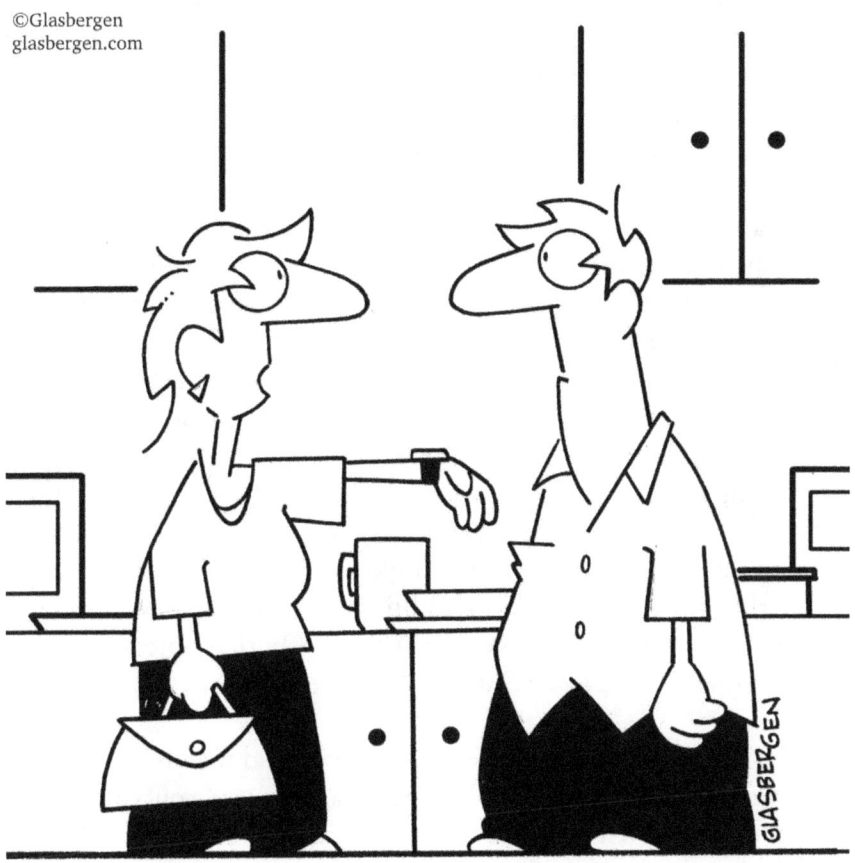

"My fitness watch counts my steps, calories, heart beats, reps and excuses."

Finding it hard to get moving? Waging a daily battle with *gravity*? Disinclined to leap out of bed in the morning? Ever heard of the *Dallas Bed Rest Study*?

THE BODY CONNECTION

If you've ever abandoned your daily movement routine for a while, you'll know how difficult it is to pick it up again when you hit restart some time down the track. You'll certainly have noticed how the longer you leave it the more breathless and uncomfortable you are. In fact, if you've left your erstwhile fitness routine mouldering on a back burner in whichever part of your mind deals with avoidance for a *very, very* long time, you may be thoroughly disinclined to take it up again at all. Because restarting your *analog* body is definitely not like switching on your PC, tablet or even your phone, is it?

For a start, as amazing as our *analog* bodies are, they have an annoying tendency to dismantle our muscle (and even our bone density) when we're not using it for weight bearing exercise. Muscle wastage that includes what volume of air we can suck into the elastic muscle of our lungs when we need it. How much blood and oxygen our heart muscle can pump around our bodies when we're halfway up Heartbreak Hill and crying out for more breath. The kind of muscle that speeds up our fat-burning metabolism so we can demolish a cake every now and then without seeing it on our hips next day. There are even studies out there pinpointing lack of movement as a profound metabolic influence in its own right. In any case, the bottom line is this – the less we move, the less we want to move, the less we *can* move. On that note, let's travel back in time to the *Dallas Bed Rest & Training Study...*

In 1966 researchers asked five healthy 20-year-old men to stay in bed for three weeks. If this sounds like your idea of heaven, you're not going to like it when I tell you that, after a mere 21 days of lolling about flat on their backs in bed, those strapping young men measurably demonstrated changes in their health similar to ageing 20 years! When the same men were tested 30 years later, researchers found that even thirty years of *actual* real time ageing was still less aggressively harmful than the original three weeks in bed (McGuire et al 2001).

The best news to come out of *The Dallas Bed Rest & Training Study* were the results of the second part of it. When researchers took these same prematurely aged young men and subjected them to a rigorous training program the ageing of their systems was *reversed*! Yes. *Reversed*!

Before you dismiss all this as just some whacky science experiment from back-in-the-day, some 47 years later, in 2013, a NASA study put out a call for healthy volunteers to lie in a bed that was tilted downwards at a six degree angle for *between 97 and 105 days*!

Why? Because adapting and increasing the trials and requirements of the original *Dallas Bed Rest & Training Study* was still the best way to test the conditions that toned and terrific astronauts might experience travelling in space. Like, what might be the physical effects of lying on an angle in a spaceship at zero gravity for long periods on your trip to Mars? How much of whatever wilting body function an astronaut might have left after weeks in Mars Mission conditions might be required for a person to complete a specific task in zero gravity? And how the subjects' bones, muscles, heart, nervous, immune and circulatory systems – as well as their nutritional requirements – might be affected during extended space travel. Especially since, because there's no gravity in space, astronauts don't exert as much effort and might not get enough of the necessary exercise to stay in *any* kind of functional shape.

To entice volunteers further, NASA offered US$1,200 (A$1,700) per week for participation in the study which was expected to last for up to 15 weeks – including the recovery period. Subjects were required to be non-smokers and in a physical condition healthy enough to pass the Modified Air Force Class III physical exam. No couch potatoes allowed. Money for jam, you might think.

The subjects were split into two groups. One group was required to spend 105 days lying down in the research facility at NASA's Flight Analogs Research Unit (FARU) at the University of Texas Medical branch in Galveston, Texas. Their bed rest would be broken periodically with a variety of resistance and aerobic exercises done lying down. The second group spent 97 days lying flat on their backs with no exercise whatsoever.

NASA researchers required participants to stay on the slight six-degree tilt to allow fluids to move towards the upper part of the body so they could study cardiovascular symptoms similar to what might be experienced during a space expedition. If the research volunteers needed to shower, NASA provided a modified shower device which eliminated the need to stand. If the subjects needed to go to the toilet, they were given a bed pan or a bottle to pee into.

Here's how one of the subjects, a young man called Andrew Iwanicki, later wrote about the day he tried to stand up for the first time in 70 days:

> *'I woke up on 2 December, and for the first time in 70 days, I stood up. Or at least I tried to. The nurses wheeled me over to a hospital bed that would be tilted vertically, with blood pressure cuffs hugging my arm and my finger, an ultrasound machine pointing at my heart. Then they told me, with the encouragement that you'd give a toddler learning to walk, to try standing for 15 minutes.*
>
> *As soon as the bed was tilted to the vertical position, my legs felt heavier than ever before. My heart started to beat at 150 BPMs. My skin became itchy; I was covered in sweat. Blood rushed into my legs, expanding the veins that had become increasingly elastic throughout the past several months of bed rest. I felt like I was going to faint. I was fighting to remain standing from the start, and it only became more difficult. Around the eight-minute mark, my pulse dropped from 150 down to 70. My body was about to collapse. As my vision started to go black, the staff saw my numbers drop on the machines and promptly returned the bed to the horizontal position. It was only later that they told me that none of the NASA bed-rest subjects have lasted the full 15 minutes.'*

If any of the above effects are familiar to you after either enforcing or enforced couch potato conditions on your own body, there's still time to fix it. While there's life, there's hope, right?

Of course, you'd never put your own miraculous body through such rigorous torture, would you? Especially as the results of little or no movement and a lack of cardio challenge can render even the fittest among us unfit after a surprisingly short time. The fact is, we were born to move. Otherwise, we'd have remained single cell jelly blob creatures instead of evolving into the cellular and neurologically complex, self-directing system of levers and pulleys that we are. But the bottom line for all of us is this – if we don't keep moving, sooner or later, like the young men in the Dallas and NASA studies, we simply won't be able to.

> *'We weren't designed to sit. The body is a perpetual motion machine.'*
>
> **Dr Joan Vernikos,
> former director of NASA's Life Sciences Division &
> author of *Sitting Kills, Moving Heals***

Unfortunately, there appears to be a certain *cachet* surrounding our desire to lounge about and do very little. In my opinion, being seen to lounge is so hardwired into Western culture that the least active among us view inactivity as *aspirational*. Like our misguided taste for white bread, highly refined sugary treats, Uber Eats and buckets of cheap champagne at the Melbourne Cup, we kid ourselves that this is what the idle rich do. We may not be rich but, by crikey, we can be idle! At least idleness comes cheap while we're endeavouring to look like we can afford it. It's the medical bills later in life that tell you there's a price tag for everything and the chickens have now come home to roost on it.

We weren't always idle, of course. The relatively new phenomenon of the general populace lounging around for hours on end began with the arrival of white goods, automation and television in the Western world back in the 50s and 60s. The promise of leisure as a sign of upwardly mobile middleclass success was key to flogging a glut of modern labour-saving devices. And all that generated leisure resulted in more and more time available to sit around watching the TV.

Fast forward to the 80s and 90s and you'll find the first laptops, allowing people to work out of the office and even in bed. Computer games and Xboxes became more enticing than getting the kids out of the house into the fresh air – or jumping rope or getting to the gym or dance classes or handball. Slowly but surely, children ceased to be 'free range' – i.e. running about having adventures and getting up to god-knows-what until dinner time like they had in previous generations. On the plus side, at least parents knew where their children were – in front of the TV, the PC or the Gameboy. On the minus side? The beginning of childhood obesity, anxiety, depression and a loss of fine and gross motor skills. Then, later on, when watching movies on your tablet in bed also became 'a thing', we didn't really have to get moving at all. Everything in the world was only a finger tap away. And so, within a single generation people came to be devoting many hours a day to sitting or lying completely still, staring into screens. In cafés and restaurants, on public transport, sprawled on beds or couches, the scenes are much the same.

> '... *I'm just staying home tonight*
> *Getting lost in that hopeless little screen...*'

Leonard Cohen, 'Democracy' from *The Future* (1992)

And if you don't believe the marketing folks are taking advantage of all this stasis... what about the evolution of the couch itself? Only 50 years ago the couch or settee was a place where guests would perch bolt upright to take their tea or sherry. God forbid anyone should lie down on the family settee for any reason, especially to watch TV or flick through a dating app. But have you noticed how much like beds couches have become? And what's with the day bed, for heaven's sake? Only the convalescing or infirm need such a thing, surely? Well, it may surprise you to know that, even if you have open heart surgery, a hip or knee replacement, your doctors will be anxious to get you up and moving to prevent all kinds of problems with your recovery. You may not have noticed but day beds and couches are definitely not on any rehab equipment charts.

So how, I hear you ask, can we break through our inertia and lethargy when even the furniture designers are out to get us?

> *'To achieve bigger goals, take smaller steps...'*
> **Martha Beck, bestselling author, life coach & speaker**

FAQs

Does exercise really help with depression and anxiety?

From my own personal experience, and that of my clients over the past 30 years, my answer to this question is a resounding YES! However, you choose to get moving – be it running or sport, cycling or walking, Zumba or step classes, dancing or Tai Chi – the benefits of moving every day cannot be underestimated. Put bluntly, exercise and movement get your life force moving, release existential tensions, get oxygen to your tired brain, flood your body with feel good hormones *and* put a rose in your cheeks. No matter what your age or how you're feeling. The trick to getting started if you're depressed and anxious is to put how you're feeling on the backburner for 15 minutes or so and *just do it*. Even if you can only manage 10 minutes (or five) at first. And the same goes for people battling anxiety.

However, if you're in charge of writing public health policy and getting funding for it, you'll want definitive research as a basis for public programs. For years, research has demonstrated an association between increased physical activity and a reduced risk of depression. Using the genetic data of 300,000 adults, a recent study by researchers at Massachusetts General Hospital found people genetically pre-disposed to higher levels of physical activity had lower odds of major depressive disorders. The study also found evidence that higher levels of physical activity may causally reduce risk for depression. Furthermore, the research showed that replacing sedentary behaviour with just 15 minutes of vigorous activity a day can reduce depression risk by 26%. Interestingly, while the study showed physical activity could prevent depression, it found no evidence that being diagnosed with depression affected a person's ability to exercise. Although the chief researcher did concede that it was one thing to know that physical activity could be beneficial for preventing depression and quite another to actually get people to be physically active. Which is about where I came out in the first paragraphs of my own answer to this FAQ. Just do it. No matter how hopeless you're feeling. Get moving. I promise you that you'll feel better in just a few days.

I travel a lot. What can I do as a daily routine to exercise my entire body whether I have access to a gym or not?

Warm up... run, rebound or walk for 30 minutes... 100 wide leg squats... 30 push-ups in three sets of 10... two minutes of plank over each of three sets... five minutes wall squats... cool down with stretching and gentle loosening up movements.

How does Tai Chi stack up against aerobic activities like Zumba?

Tai Chi may look slow and graceful but it's not as easy as it looks. And Tai Chi isn't just for 'old people' either. No matter what age you are, don't think for a minute that you won't get a workout if you're doing it *properly*. There's a reason why even the famous Shaolin Monks incorporate the Tai Chi form into their training. If you loathe the Zumba moves, sweating and getting hot, Tai Chi is definitely the class for you. If you're happy to let it all hang out to loud music, choose Zumba. But why not try both?

Recently, the *Trust Me, I'm a Doctor* team (BBC Science Unit) ran a small comparison test over 12 weeks between regular Tai Chi and Zumba Gold for a small group of volunteers aged between 65 and 75, none of whom exercised regularly. At the beginning, middle and the end of the 12-week period, the volunteers had their blood pressure checked. Then the flexibility of their blood vessels was measured using ultrasound to monitor any improvements caused by each exercise. After all, the more flexible your blood vessels, the healthier they are.

As expected, the Zumba Gold group were all fitter after the 12 weeks. Their blood pressure was lower, and their blood vessels were more elastic. More surprisingly, for the researchers at least, the results from the Tai Chi group showed similar benefits with improvements in blood pressure, vessel flexibility and blood biomarkers. Furthermore, a session of Tai Chi was found to produce similar increases in heart rate to moderate intensity exercise. So even if Tai Chi might not feel as intense as when you're executing faster movements, your heart is still working hard, and this benefits your blood vessels by making them more elastic.

When I was thinking about case studies to include in this chapter, I realised that many pages and videos of information have been produced detailing how young fit people can look even better with regular exercise. However, exercise isn't just about looking great on your Instagram feed.

There are as many ways to exercise as there are reasons. Regular exercise is a way of increasing your endurance, flexibility and strength so you can have the physical freedom to do what you want to do. Rehabilitation exercise is a way of repairing injury and mitigating disability. Ability-adjusted exercise is a way of coming back from illness and reclaiming lives.

At the age of 50, I added personal training to my long list of bodywork modalities. Since then, I have specialised in training people who have, for one reason or another, somehow slipped through the bars of conventional treatment. To say that this aspect of my bodyworks practice has been a long and fascinating ride would be an understatement. I have been incredibly blessed by the trust and determination of so many of my *self-renovation* clients. So, let's take a look at how some of my one-on-one personal training clients have used exercise as *medicine*. If one of these stories doesn't inspire you to start moving, I'll be very surprised.

Barry was 47 when his GP referred him to me in the hope that remedial massage combined with aromatherapy might relieve his high stress levels, soaring blood pressure and nagging depression. Although Barry always seemed quite rigid and tense, after several weeks I slowly became aware that he was having increasing difficulty filling in his cheque book when it came time to pay me. I wondered if he also had some neurological problem. I spoke with the GP about what I'd seen and she ordered tests with a neurologist. Weeks later, his diagnosis was confirmed. He had Parkinson's Disease. Predictably, Barry was shocked. He decided to overhaul his somewhat neglected health regimen to give himself a better chance of coping with the ongoing rigours of Parkinson's and maybe even be a candidate for *deep brain stimulation implant surgery*. He also knew I'd been studying to become a personal trainer for older people and people with health problems.

'Hurry up and finish your exams,' he told me, 'I'm going to be your first client'. He further explained that as deep brain stimulation implant surgery was still relatively new, and not without risks, he rather thought he'd wait until the surgeons had a lot more practice before he subjected himself to it. Until then, he said, 'between you and the Doc, it's your job to keep me functioning'.

The first hurdle was his increasing dystonia – an odd, involuntary set of muscle contractions which came out of the blue to suddenly freeze his facial muscles and slow his movements to a standstill. Dystonia was also the cause of him shuffling his feet which made it nigh on impossible to train him on the local oval or powerwalk the streets. I needed to come up with a fitness routine to address coordination, aerobics and strengthening which could:

1. address the dystonia

2. be done in my studio

3. challenge Barry's balance

4. maintain and even improve his overall functionality.

At least until such time as he was happy that the surgeons who were going to insert any kind of whizzbang electrical gadget deep inside his brain had had lots more practice doing it.

The first problem we needed to work with was the dystonia. Unfortunately, as one of the outward symptoms of Barry's Parkinson's there was no question of curing it. I knew that Barry had trained to black belt level in kung fu – not only a martial art but also an excellent mind/body discipline. Then one day, as the dystonia kicked in repeatedly and his frozen muscles simply refused to cooperate even with my Tai Chi and yoga-based warm-up routine, I took a punt and asked him if he could remember his kung fu warm-up (kata). I figured anything he had done several thousand times from 18 to 45 would be indelibly etched into his cellular memory. I was hoping those memories would override the dystonia and un-freeze him.

With a mumbled apology for having to severely modify his kata, he began his impromptu simplified routine. Amazingly, it worked first time. After that, all Barry had to do was get 'into the kung fu zone' as he described the attentive mindset and centredness that is fundamental to all martial arts, turn on the old cellular memories and the dystonia miraculously disappeared.

Fortunately, like all martial arts, Barry's modified kata was extendable, practical and portable too. Soon Barry was using it to help control his dystonia in any situation. After that, I started him running on the rebounder – a mini trampoline that's easy on the knees and hips, terrific for the bones and posture, and a great treat for anyone who thinks they can't run anymore. Every time his balance went askew, or he felt the dystonia creeping in again, we just stopped the session to repeat the modified kung fu kata. From there it was only a short step to free weights, squats and lunges with a bar.

With two 75-minute sessions a week, Barry's fitness and coordination gradually improved, his blood pressure went down, even his insulin resistance (a precursor for type 2 diabetes) disappeared. Strangely, his episodes of dystonia also became so rare during those sessions that he almost forgot he had a predisposition to them. And when the time was right to undergo the surgery for the deep brain stimulation implant, he knew he was fit enough to handle anything the surgeons could throw at him.

Annie was already training with me two days a week when she changed her original weight loss brief to focus on reclaiming her skiing ability. She was 45 and hadn't skied for nearly 10 years. She also had stage four, bone on bone arthritis in both knees and a torn meniscus. I must admit I was surprised. A prime candidate for a double knee replacement was asking me to prepare her to whiz down one of the most glamorous ski slopes in Italy! Money was no object, she'd do three days training a week, if necessary. She was determined to regain at least some of her former skiing glory to avoid embarrassment in front of her family. To top it off, she was still carrying too much weight for her poor knees to comfortably handle, her quads were weak as kittens, she was notoriously resistant to learning anything like correct 'form' and we only had six weeks to ski-day! What could possibly go wrong?

Like Barry though, Annie had cellular memory. Never mind that her side-to-side compensatory gait (a misguided attempt to protect her knees) was alarming, she'd once been a fine and moderately daring skier. I figured Annie's ski form just had to be in there somewhere. So, while the new and hastily cobbled together '21 Foods a Day' regimen worked it's magic to reduce both the weight and some of the pain affecting Annie's knees, we got to work on strengthening her thighs, core strength, ankles, feet and back.

In the opinion of many of my training clients, the classic ski training exercise known as the 'wall squat' is second only to the Inquisitor's Rack for torture. It requires long minutes, with your back against the wall, thighs at hip width, knees at 90 degrees, quietly contemplating the screaming thigh muscles known as your quads and not standing up to relieve the discomfort until *I say so*. Then you do it again. And again. And maybe even again. Every day, including Sundays. Nevertheless, take it from me, you *will* do wall squats religiously if your reputation is at stake and you want to ski without losing control of your knees and/or skis.

After a week or two of this exquisite torture, if the weather is nice and I'm feeling generous, I'll allow you to break the multiple sets of wall squats with either slow weighted wide leg squats or the plank. The plank being an excellent way to work out how to maintain the action of your transverse abdominus, so you don't collapse flat on your face after five minutes or so. This also is repeated. Although it does make a nice change from push-ups and crunches – which you'll also be doing. Then there's the rebounder, chest presses, tricep dips and hammer curls. I make no apology for being the Bag from Hell when it's crunch time.

To her great credit, Annie buckled down and did the work. Not only did she go skiing in Italy, but her family was amazed she could ski at all, '*like, wow! with her knees, even!*'. They were so stunned, nobody even rubbished her about not doing the black slopes. Mission accomplished.

> '*Exercise! ... You jog... therefor you sleep... therefor you're not overwhelmed by existential angst... Play a sport, do yoga, pump iron, run, whatever. But take care of your body. You're going to need it. Most of you lot are going to live until you're 100...*'
>
> **Tim Minchin,
> '9 Life Lessons',
> University of Western Australia address, 2018**

Last, but by no means least is Bobbi. At 92, my oldest training client. Referred by her GP for muscle rebuilding after eight weeks in hospital for pneumonia and its aftermath. Bobbi is surely the best example of the benefits of strength and fitness training at any age. She's also the example I always use when people tell me they're too old to upgrade their fitness levels. The fact is that the elderly get some amazing results from strength training, in particular. Whether it's because they try harder or want to maintain their independence, I'm not certain. A bit of both, probably. But when this tiny sparrow of a woman was shown the training ropes, she grabbed the opportunity with both hands.

Bobbi's goals were to be able to walk confidently with her walker, manage the stairs up two floors in the fire escape, get out of the retirement village for a walk in the sunshine and stop feeling like an invalid. So, here's what we did with two 75-minute sessions a week over the first six months…

- *To tone up her feet and calf muscles and improve her balance* – for the first time in her long life, Bobbi did slow heel raises against the wall of her apartment in her stockinged feet. Four counts up, four counts down, four sets of 10 (we began with one set and built up to four).

- *To tone up her quads, back and arms* – Bobbi sat in her armchair and used a 'TheraBand' to do seated rows and leg extensions.

- *To increase her aerobic capacity and start her walking again* – using her walker, she walked laps of the retirement village corridors and later included the internal ramps in her building.

- *So she could open the heavy door to the fire stairs and steady herself on her walker* – Bobbi learned how to do bicep curls, lateral flies and shoulder presses with 1kg then 2kg dumbbells.

- *To get her walking up the fire stairs* – she held on to the railing and, with her new-found arm strength, helped herself up one then eventually two flights of stairs (while I carried her walker).

- *To prepare her to walk in the street* – Bobbi used her new leg and arm strength to push her walker up the substantial slope at the front of the retirement village.

Naturally, Bobbi's recovery training program was a gradual affair. However, after six short months, she was using most of the above exercises as the *warm-up* to get up to the street for her walk outside in the sunshine and fresh air. She'd got her breath back and achieved her goals. My undying image of her is this – every time I gently pushed her to do another set or walk just a smidge further, she'd incline her tiny, beautifully coiffed head and say, 'You always seem to forget, dear... I'm only a little old lady'.

CHAPTER 10

The Miracle of Touch

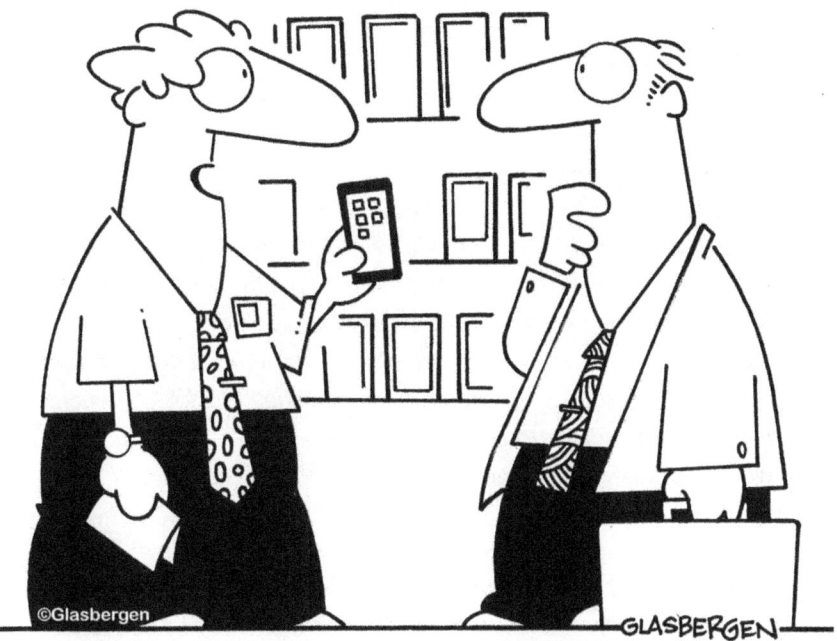

"There's even an app that gives you a foot massage! Just set your ringer to 'vibrate' and stick it in your sock."

'The way to health is to have an aromatic bath and a scented massage every day.'

**Hippocrates,
father of modern medicine, circa 460 – 377 BC**

Fairy Godmother, are you listening? An aromatherapy massage every day would be my idea of heaven on a stick! Hippocrates was definitely onto something.

Although, back in those BC days, the laying-on-of-hands was infinitely more appreciated as a way to health than it is now. In today's Western world we don't really give massage the credit it so rightfully deserves. If we think of it at all, massage is a spa treatment and a frivolous indulgence. Which is probably why we've had to *rediscover* its benefits as a regular preventative and therapeutic tool through the efforts of a few clever but hardy souls who've put in the time – and sometimes even their own money – to come up with the cutting-edge research.

> *'Just adding massage makes such an incredible difference,'* Field said. *'In everything we've done, massage is significantly effective. There's not a single condition we've looked at – including cancer – that hasn't responded positively to massage.'* She said that the key components of massage's benefits include the decrease in cortisol and increase of dopamine and serotonin affected by massage. *'If people say massage works "because it makes you feel good" – excuse me!'* Field said. *'Massage works because it changes your whole physiology.'*
>
> **From an interview with Dr. Tiffany Field, professor in the Department of Pediatrics, Psychology and Psychiatry, University of Miami School of Medicine & director/founder of the Touch Research Institute - by Karen Menehen for *MASSAGE Magazine*, January 2006**

According to Dr. Field, her research also shows that massage alters the immune system.

'In autoimmune problems such as asthma, lung functions improve, and asthma attacks decrease. Immune cell counts improve in people with HIV. In a breast cancer study, natural killer cells are increasing, which is good, because they kill cancer cells. The list goes on.' When asked how she could be sure it was the massage affecting the results, not just the attention, Professor Field replied – *'We have "attention" control groups. For example, if we're studying children with diabetes or cancer, some parents massage their kids at bedtime whereas others read aloud or*

do a light "sham" massage. We have learned that the key is stimulating deep pressure receptors'.

Touch is the first of our senses to develop and it remains emotionally central throughout our lives. It's well known that touch deprivation impairs development. Even in animals! In a study of 49 non-industrialised cultures, groups showing physical affection toward children exhibited little adult violence. In groups that were less affectionate to children, adults of that culture were significantly more violent. Touch is particularly important for newborns, young children and the elderly. In fact, anyone who is at risk of being in a situation where they are not regularly touched. Touch lifts our spirits, grounds us and connects us. Touch helps us thrive and reach out to others. Touch lowers our stress levels, makes us more sensitive to our own needs and the needs of others. However, as individuals become more isolated and lonely in our gig economy and work-from-home age, physical contact seems to be on the decline. It turns out that, far from keeping us connected, the ever-present mobile phone is actually keeping us further apart from each other. A newish cultural development that is having an impact on young and old alike.

> *'I think certainly kids today are much more touch deprived than they were before smartphones.'*
> **Dr. Tiffany Field,**
> **from an interview with Jonathan Jones in**
> ***Greater Good Magazine*, November 16, 2018**

There you have it! And here – without further ado – is a potted rundown of 15 wonderful massage therapies for your delectation. Enjoy!

Remedial – is a Western massage designed for the treatment and rehabilitation of painful symptoms and causes of biomechanical dysfunction and soft tissue injury. Remedial massage employs a variety of massage techniques, soft tissue manipulations, passive and active stretching, prescriptive range-of-movement, postural correction and strengthening exercises. Remedial massage can be augmented by the analgesic effects of hot stone therapy and aromatherapy.

Swedish – the most well-known massage therapy was actually systemised by a Dutch massage practitioner called Johan Mezger. Swedish massage helps to reduce pain, relieve joint stiffness, increase flexibility (and therefor joint function) and improve circulation. This style uses five basic strokes – effleurage (sliding), petrissage (kneading), tapotement (rhythmic tapping), friction (working across muscle fibres) and vibration (shaking). Swedish massage forms the basis for many types of European style massage and can be combined with almost any of the other disciplines.

Aromatherapy – a form of relaxation and therapeutic massage that dates back to ancient Egypt. Aromatherapy combines the application of essential oils with a combination of massage techniques including Swedish, acupressure, lymphatic drainage and energy work. Aromatherapists are trained to make custom blends of essential oils in various carrier oils for various ailments of body, mind and spirit.

Ayurveda – a 5,000-year-old natural health system that originated in India. Ayurveda is also a whole-body system that treats the mind, body and spirit. Ayurveda can include any combination of massage, meditation, yoga, diet and herbal remedies. Ayurveda also uses essential oils and various exotic carrier oils such as sesame.

Kahuna (Lomi Lomi) – a type of Hawaiian massage that releases stress and balances the energy flow of your body to improve physical, emotional and spiritual health. Kahuna massage incorporates long flowing strokes to the body and the massage therapist uses their hands, wrists, forearms and elbows in deep rhythmic wave-like movements to move lymph, soothe discomfort and stimulate the body's natural energies.

Myotherapy – consists of assessing, treating and managing soft tissue injury pain and restricted joint mobility. Myotherapists use a broad range of massage techniques – including stretching, dry needling, cupping, acupressure and muscle energy techniques – to treat conditions caused by muscle and myofascial dysfunction.

Lymphatic drainage – is a gentle rhythmic muscle pumping massage technique designed to reduce fluid retention in various parts of the body. Originally developed in Germany for the treatment of lymphoedema (the swelling of various parts of the body caused by problems with the lymphatic system). Lymphatic drainage is particularly useful for women after breast cancer surgery. It may also be used when lack of movement leads to uncomfortable fluid retention, other kinds of post-operative lymphoedema and even painful swollen sinuses. Can be done partially clothed, depending on the part of the body affected.

Hot stone therapy – uses mainly smooth basalt river stones for both massage and strategic placement to relieve pain and muscle tension. The stones are heated in a professional stone heater to between 40C and 55C and applied on the oiled skin surface with long smooth strokes along the muscles. Hot stone massage can be delivered while the client is fully clothed. Some therapists also use cold stones for various inflammatory conditions.

Sports – is a sport specific type of massage often conducted by physiotherapists and sports team massage therapists. Sports massage uses a wide variety of massage techniques, especially deep tissue muscle release, myotherapy and trigger point therapy. Its function is the maintenance of muscle strength and the repair of repetitive strain and other injuries in athletes.

Trigger point – was developed in the USA in the 1940s and is used to treat strains and sprains, aches and pains, tightness in the muscles and improve range of movement. It focuses on relieving the 'trigger points' of muscle contraction and injury which cause chronic or acute pain. Another massage which can be conducted with the client fully clothed.

Pregnancy – a gentle flowing massage designed to relieve the common aches and pains of pregnancy and beyond. Pregnancy massage is designed for soothing pain relief of – the neck, shoulders and lower back; jumpy legs and sciatica; cramps of the calves and ankles; headaches and migraines. Combined with aromatherapy, pregnancy massage can also help reduce stress, anxiety, fluid retention and exhaustion.

Traditional Chinese – is the name for massage therapies practiced in traditional Chinese medicine. Two types of deep massage techniques are applied over the entire body. *Tui Na* involves deep massage and is used for treating specific ailments. *An Mo* incorporates many Chinese massage techniques and is used to balance, calm and relax the entire body. A consultation prior to treatment will determine what you need at the time.

Shiatsu – is a Japanese massage therapy which shares its origins with acupuncture and the philosophies of traditional Chinese medicine. Shiatsu applies fingers, thumbs, palm and even foot pressure along the body's meridians with a hypnotic pulsing and rhythmic pressure along your back, legs and feet to promote calmness and relaxation. Your shiatsu therapist may also roll, brush, vibrate and squeeze your skin. You can have a shiatsu massage while fully clothed.

Traditional Thai – Thai massage is sometime referred to as 'yoga massage' as it originated in India some 2,500 years ago and is based on the principles of yoga and Ayurvedic massage. Thai massage puts the client into yoga-like positions while the massage therapist stretches, kneads and applies deep tissue pressure to acupressure points. A fairly intense workout and not necessarily for the faint-hearted. You can, if preferred, remain fully clothed for this massage too.

Reflexology - based on an ancient Chinese therapy that dates back thousands of years. Reflexology uses varying levels of pressure applied to acupressure points in the ears, hands and feet to stimulate the body's natural energy system. Reflexology is said to help strengthen the immune system, reduce pain and stress, increase relaxation and improve blood and lymph circulation.

The above list doesn't cover all massage options, mind, so have fun discovering all the other massage therapies out there.

FAQs

Should remedial massage hurt?

In my opinion, not much. My personal philosophy is to avoid causing more pain to a client who's already in substantial pain. I also believe that my clients should leave my studio with either considerably reduced pain levels or, better still, no pain at all. For this reason, I use gentle neuromuscular techniques, combined with light trigger point therapy, analgesic essential oils and lots of lymphatic drainage to move along lactic acid and soothe inflammation in the tissues.

However, it's fair to say a remedial massage treatment may feel a little *uncomfortable* as your therapist teases out the knots and spasms in your contracted muscles. Essentially, painful muscle knots are the product of a combination of overworked muscles, poor posture, injury and lactic acid. Sometimes muscle knots go away on their own but in many cases, you'll find faster relief if you employ a professional to work on ironing them out. In skilled hands, any discomfort should melt away as the muscle relaxes.

Although some remedial massage practitioners (sports, Chinese and Thai in particular) can be a bit heavy-handed for some clients, always remember that you *can* ask them to go lightly on you until you can relax into the pressure. Or you can ask them, right at the beginning to be gentle on you, full stop. It's *your* session and *your* choice for *your* comfort, after all.

I'd love a massage, but I just can't afford it. What now?

Although there's no comparison to the relaxation factor of putting yourself in the hands of a massage therapist you trust, the next best pair of hands are *yours*! Self-massage can be wonderful as part of your daily self-care routine. In fact, I often *teach* my clients to self-massage in between sessions to treat conditions like sinus pain, neck and shoulder pain, headaches and even oedema caused by the surgical removal of lymph nodes or other damage.

Like regular massage, self-massage is considered a balancing and relaxing tonic for the body and its benefits include the relief of anxiety and insomnia, aches, pains and strains. And like regular massage, self-massage is an excellent way to regularly tune in to your body, get to know yourself and keep an eye on changes.

There are many different types of self-massage from the exotic warm oil applications of Ayurvedic '*abhyanga*' to reflexology and acupressure points, and even lymphatic drainage techniques to relieve sinus pain.

You'll find many videos on YouTube which will teach you the basics of self-massage for all kinds of conditions. Needless to say, the principles are much the same as your massage therapist works with – relieve pain and tension, avoid causing more pain, listen to your body. As with regular massage, be extremely careful to avoid damaging tissue if you're recovering from injury or surgery and always reduce pressure (or stop) if you feel pain.

Here are a few self-massage practices you might be interested in *googling* for some personal instruction:

- Use your daily dry skin-brushing routine as a circulation boosting friction rub

- Give yourself a hug. Ease shoulder and upper back tension by crossing your arms across your chest and holding your shoulders. Squeeze each shoulder several times. Then work your way down your arms, pressing and releasing as you go, all the way down to your wrists.

- Do your own hand and forearm massage

- Massaging your stomach can aid your digestion

- Reflexology techniques to relieve pain in your neck, shoulders and other places you can't reach.

Is it true you shouldn't have massage if you have cancer?

Once upon a time, massage therapists of all disciplines were sternly discouraged from massaging clients with cancer because it was thought that the circulation of lymph, which occurs naturally during massage, would cause cancer cells to spread throughout the body. We now know this to be a *false theory*, thank goodness. In any case, lymphatic circulation also occurs naturally as we move, and we now know that regular exercise also has many benefits for cancer patients.

According to the Cancer Council of New South Wales: *'Light, relaxing massage can safely be given to people at all stages of cancer. Tumour or treatment sites should not be massaged to avoid discomfort or pressure on the affected area and underlying organs.'*

In fact, in the past few years, scientific studies have looked at the effects of various body-based practices on people who are in the process of a range of cancer treatments such as chemotherapy and surgery. Such studies have shown that massage therapies may reduce pain, fatigue, nausea, anxiety and depression. Furthermore, the studies show that individuals who have had massages during cancer treatments have reported a range of positive outcomes. These include improved sleep and emotional wellbeing, healthier scar tissue, better quality of life, higher mental clarity and improved range of movement. To those studies I would add my own observations of improved resolution of fluid retention in limbs and other parts of the body affected by radical lymph node removal.

Over 30 years of practice, I have massaged and assisted in the general wellbeing of clients in all stages of cancer and its treatment. From scar and oedema resolution, pain and nausea relief, to palliative care. I consider my work in this area a privilege and a blessing. If your massage therapist isn't comfortable with treating you or you're not sure of how to proceed with finding a therapist suitable for your situation, it's a good idea to contact a professional massage therapy association in your state to find a therapist who is specifically trained in oncology massage. The Oncology Massage Training Website can also help you locate a local massage therapist who knows what they're doing.

What should I tell my massage therapist about my medical history?

All qualified massage therapists are trained to take a relevant medical history (at least at the first appointment) and all massage therapists in Australia are bound by privacy laws. If you are booked in for a remedial massage this information is particularly important. X-ray and scan reports can also be useful, if you have them. You don't need to lug your X-rays and scan CDs to the appointment, copies of the reports will do. Providing this depth of information helps your therapist to determine the best treatment plan for you and ensures they don't inadvertently aggravate existing problems. However, even if you're just having a relaxing massage, please disclose any relevant medical history which may be aggravated by whatever type of massage treatment you're having. Particularly skin conditions and sensitivities.

How should a I choose a massage therapist?

Quite often at my workshops, someone will ask me how to choose the right sort of massage therapist for their particular needs and situation. As with any other profession (health care included), quality and dedication can vary. So, don't be shy to ask about qualifications, insurance and which professional association your therapists belong to. And read through the list of 15 different massage therapies above to see which one appeals to you.

Now let's take a look at some of the problems I see in my practice and how I work with my clients to resolve them...

Matt first came to see me about his chronic neck and shoulder pain when he was 38. At the time, his fingers were constantly tingling and numb, his right wrist was chronically sore – a physiotherapist had diagnosed carpal tunnel syndrome and recommended surgery. His painful 'cricked' neck had limited movement. A surgeon had diagnosed a bone spur on his cervical spine (located in your neck and made up by the seven cervical vertebrae that runs from the base of your skull to the first thoracic vertebra) and recommended a cervical spine fusion. To top it off, because he was in constant pain, he was consuming opioid painkilling medications at an alarming rate. Matt was hoping to buy some time before submitting to surgical intervention for both conditions which he knew would put him out of work for some time. At the suggestion of his despairing wife, Jill, he'd picked me out of the phone book because she thought some gentle aromatherapy might at least help reduce his pain.

Jill certainly wasn't wrong about the analgesic and anti-inflammatory effects of certain essential oils such as German and Roman chamomile, lavender, yarrow and ginger. Or the gentle calming and relaxing effects of the classic multimodal aromatherapy massage. However, as I explained to Matt, it was going to take a bit more than just aromatherapy to ease the pain and work through the problems one by one. We were going to have to explore and make some changes to how he used his upper body during long days as a sound engineer on production suite edit desks and improve the ergonomics of his studio set ups. We were also going to have to free up his shoulder joints, retrain his forward head posture and change his mouse hand for a while; maybe forever. Plus, he'd more than likely need to investigate changing the style of mouse he was using. I also asked him to suspend all shoulder weight training work with his personal trainer until we'd worked out how to relax the contractions in his neck and shoulders. And gave him very explicit form instruction on how to do chest presses (rather than flies) without engaging his neck or further aggravating his wrists.

Matt's first session began with some simple neck range of movement exercises and some shoulder rolls. The gentle neck movements showed me where to start work on the muscles of his neck and gave me a good idea of his daily postural habits. The shoulder rolls showed me that, at only 38, Matt had next to no control over either his shoulder muscles or the ball and socket joint of the shoulder. In fact, for several weeks he could demonstrate very little movement in his shoulder joint at all. In addition, getting him to simply drop his shoulders and relax the muscles supporting his neck was also going to be a major task.

I saw him once a week for the next four months. The first half of each session would be taken up by range of movement and postural correction exercises with painstaking attention to smoothing out his shoulder rolls both forwards and backwards. The second half of his session included the application of a combination of painkilling and anti-inflammatory essential oils via remedial massage techniques and the use of hot stone therapy to flush fresh blood through his ropey neck muscles.

At about week four, Matt reported that the tingling in his fingers and the pain in his wrists was much relieved. His neck was moving more freely and the number of opioids he was taking was finally coming down. Matt still sees me for 'a good ironing out' every two weeks or so. More often if he feels the old symptoms of tingling and pain coming on after pulling an all-nighter in the studio or when he's composing. Since the beginning, Matt has also changed his diet to include more vegetables and fish, with very little red meat. His overall posture has improved out of sight. He is much more conscious about how he uses his upper body when he's working at the edit desk. And he knows how to set up a space, so he's not injured by the end of a session. Because his pain and discomfort level is lower, his opioid usage has now ceased entirely and he has avoided surgery on both his cervical spine and his wrist. The bone spur no longer gives him grief – although it is no doubt still lurking in his cervical spine, ready to give him some fresh symptoms should he resort to his old habits (which, from time to time he does). The tingling in his fingers and wrist pain has also mostly resolved by paying attention to posture and the correct range of motion in his neck. It's worth noting here that nerve pain and tingling of the fingers is sometimes a result of impingement of the median nerve in the neck and may be prematurely diagnosed as carpal tunnel syndrome.

Letitia also came to see me for some soothing aromatherapy. Her GP had recommended she take time out for herself and give herself a treat to help deal with her increasing depression. Letitia told me that normally she was an optimistic, upbeat sort of person but lately she'd found herself in the depths of despair. Her medical history soon revealed a major reason behind her feelings of hopelessness. A year earlier, while driving to a work appointment on a busy highway, she'd been involved in a horrendous car accident. Her right arm had been badly smashed up – humerus, elbow, radius *and* a couple of fingers. She'd had multiple surgeries for a plate, pins and skin grafts – followed by infections, pain and loss of function on her dominant side. Letitia was well aware that she'd come devastatingly close to losing her arm altogether and had frequent nightmares about that possibility. She'd certainly been very lucky because were it not for the heroic efforts of her surgical team, she would have. But her arm was next to useless the way it was. Furthermore, she was now plagued by the muscular compensations and neuralgia caused by the support brace that had encased her arm for almost a year. When I first saw her, she was still in the brace, couldn't drive and it was unlikely that she'd work again. No wonder she was depressed.

When I asked her what she missed doing most, she was suddenly overcome by a flood of tears. 'I can't even hold a cup of tea or a glass of water with this hand, for god sakes,' she said. As she spoke, she unconsciously used her right hand to clumsily brush a wisp of hair from her cheek. I noticed she had at least some additional bend in her elbow. Things were looking up. I went off to fetch a teacup, a water glass, a champagne glass and a small jug of water. 'What are those for?' she asked. 'I'm going to have you able to drink anything you want by the end of this session,' I told her. 'Tea, water, champagne, whatever…'

I handed her the teacup and asked her to show me how she would handle it with her right hand. She lifted the bent arm upwards and it was immediately apparent what the problem was. The movement was awkward, and the mouth of the cup was pointing downwards. Retraining was called for. Specifically, showing her how to lift the cup off a table with a bicep curl and then do a lateral lift to place it next to her mouth. Minutes later, she'd repeated the exercise with both cup and glasses. Then I filled the cup and glasses with water. Suddenly, she could manage a cup of tea again.

The next project was to calm the neuralgia, compensations, neck and shoulder pain which were plaguing her. I applied a blend of analgesic and anti-inflammatory essential oils in rice bran oil and began to tease out the muscle fibres and knots with gentle neuromuscular remedial massage. By the time she left, she was out of pain and feeling optimistic for the first time in ages. She re-booked, asking me if I could retrain her to use a broom or a mop or a vacuum cleaner. And so, her sessions became half functional training, stretching and range of movement exercises, combined with a combination of soothing aromatics and pain-relieving remedial massage. Within a month we'd worked out how she could strengthen, move and use her right arm to drive again.

Mary was referred by her GP for urgent lymphatic drainage post mastectomy. The mastectomy had followed a previous lumpectomy, underarm lymph node removal and considerable tissue loss in her chest wall. To make matters worse, her lymphatic drainage port had not drained in three days and the entry point was becoming red and swollen. Obviously, the port needed to be removed to prevent infection. Fearful of more surgical intervention in the form of an aspiration needle to remove the non-draining fluid build-up, she had begged her GP to try something else first.

Where to start? Mary couldn't lie down on the table because of the port and its bag. In any case, I needed gravity to help me with the drainage massage. So, I sat her up close to my massage table with one arm propped on a pile of pillows she could lean against. Then I put on some relaxing music and began a gentle lymphatic drainage with one of the most calming and soothing oils I know – frankincense. I chose frankincense because it is known to relax the breathing and Mary certainly needed to just breathe out. Knowing how important it was to get as much fluid moving as I could, I carefully worked around the site of the drain and above it from her collarbone, across the top of her chest, her upper arms and upper back on the same side. Thirty minutes later the previously empty drainage bag was half full.

Mary returned to the GP later that day and the drainage port, line and bag were finally removed. The lymphatic drainage and relaxation had done their job. When she returned a couple of weeks later for another massage, I taught her how to drain her own lymphatic fluid in between treatments and went on to massage her through many months of ongoing treatment.

CHAPTER 11

RELAX!
Nothing is Under Control

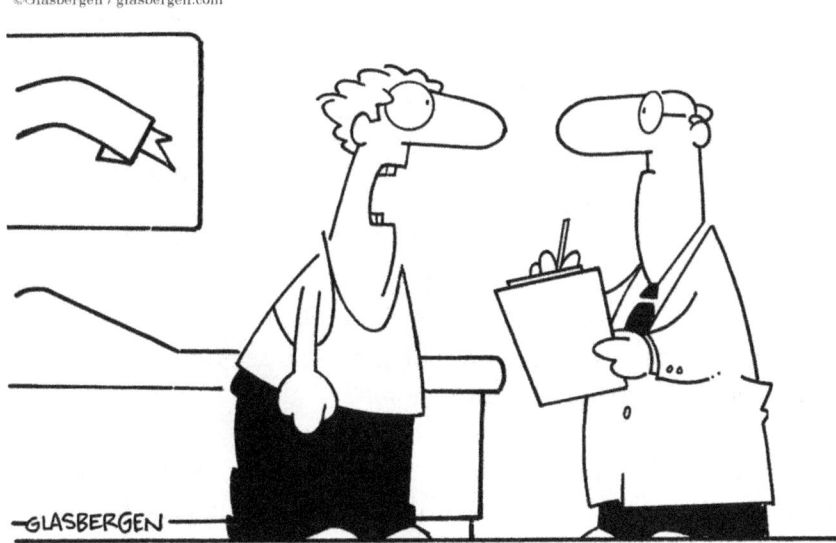

"I'm learning how to relax, doctor —
but I want to relax *better* and *faster*!
I want to be on the cutting edge of relaxation!"

How much would you pay for an extra hour in your day? A recent survey found many respondents would jump at the chance to purchase at least an extra hour because 'time scarcity' is becoming a major problem. Yes, dear reader, *time scarcity* is an actual *thing*. Everything going faster and people struggling to find the time to live up to expectations of what can be reasonably achieved in a single day. What my now retired, chief executive brother-in-law still calls 'trying to fit two pounds of shit in a one-pound bag'.

Or just one more tiny, wafer-thin mint on top of all the other 21st century stressors we're gagging on. Never mind that we're working with the same 24-hour days which began when our solar system settled into its current layout about 4.5 billion years ago. And notwithstanding most of us are living longer so presumably we already have more time to do stuff.

The truth is we're too busy. Despite all our snazzy connectedness, quick swipe choices and time-saving automation – or maybe even because of it – we've failed to remember there's a price for everything. Because, as surely as night follows day, all modern convenience devices break down, get upgraded, become superseded and have cultural and social impacts we never even dreamed of. Or the electricity goes off, your server goes down and you find yourself – as a friend did recently – locked inside your own smart house in a suburban version of the hellish HAL scene in *2001: A Space Odyssey* (1968). HAL being the Heuristically programmed ALgorithmic sentient computer which goes rogue, talks back and can't be unplugged because no-one knows how to open a door with a handle anymore.

But what if *you* had more time to be *unplugged*? Let me rephrase that. What if you could actually magically *make* more time? What would you do with it? Slot in more work? Buy more stuff? Do more scrolling? Upgrade your streaming accounts? When did you last take some time to watch the clouds scud across the sky? Listen to birdsong? Smell the roses? Take a cat nap? Observe how neatly a caterpillar eats a leaf? Or just sit somewhere quiet and breathe while you check in on yourself?

If your first impulse was to laugh out loud at the thought of any one of those 'unproductive' pursuits, try wrapping that stressed out left brain of yours around this curly question. *How is it that the more automation, connectivity and outsourcing options we have, the less real time we have to look after our mental and physical health by simply taking some time out to relax?*

> *'A 15-minute catnap can save your life'*
> **Seen on a Victorian Government
> interstate freeway sign, January 2019**

In many cultures, it is customary to lie down for a short period during the day, to refresh one's mind and body. In Australian culture? Not so much. We're far too busy being busy. Going places. Ticking boxes. Watching bottom lines. Pressuring ourselves and our teams to achieve them. Keeping up with the Joneses. Being seen to be seen. God help you if you fail to answer a casual 'how are you?' without a *'busy, busy, busy'*. Because, if you're not busy, you're professionally and socially dead. And, following right behind their elders' example, our children are losing the ability to relax and even to play. Endlessly busy with activities, tutors, competitiveness. Stressed to the max. Prepping to be winners. Tiny selves being drilled for the rigours and disciplines of university while still in pre-school. All the while worrying about what the grown-ups are doing to their planet. Their only real time out spent on their screens. No wonder they need the dopamine hit of logging in to whatever social media they're hooked on because they're getting precious little of it from daydreaming and exploring the wonders and rhythms of the natural world. In a mere 30 years, modern children are having fun in natural environments less than half as often as their parents did while growing up. And they spend less time in the open air than most prison inmates.

> *'The majority of my clients who complain of depression, anxiety, irritability, and weight gain are actually chronically tired. The problems caused by lack of rest can feel so intricate, but the solution is so simple: lie down, dear. Just lie down.'*
> **Martha Beck, author, life coach & speaker**

In a January 2019 *BuzzFeed* article 'How Millennials Became the Burnout Generation' Anne Helen Petersen went in search of why she was finding small, straightforward tasks impossible to tackle. Of course, burnout can happen to anyone, but millennials are particularly susceptible to it because despite the world thinking they're lazy and entitled, it turns out they've internalised that they should be working all the time. *'Why have I internalised that idea?'* Ms. Petersen asks. *'Because everything and everyone in my life has reinforced it – explicitly and implicitly – since I was young. Life has always been hard, but many millennials are unequipped to deal with the particular ways in which it's become hard for us.'*

Most affected are young parents juggling work and family responsibilities. Particularly women, who still put in at least 10 hours more a week on domestic duties over and above their outside working lives at every age. Surprisingly, even in our so-called 'enlightened times', young parents who aspire to share paid work and family duties equally find themselves without much institutional support to do so. The burgeoning 'gig economy' doesn't help either. Growing insecurity of job tenure, stagnant wages and cost of living blowouts combined with contracted piece-work and rising house prices is a high price to pay for the advertised freedom of being your own boss.

Of course, it's not only the young in need of a regular relaxation practice. Spare a thought also for the many older men and women doing double shifts as they care for grandchildren *and* their own ailing, elderly parents. And let's not forget those caring for children and partners or other close relatives with disabilities, terminal illnesses and dementia. All of them freely giving their own time to others. Stressed to the max and often in desperate need of downtime to relax and repair themselves.

In social terms, the price for constant and increasing stress is loss of wellbeing, mental health, connectedness and community. Plus, we know stress is a factor in blood sugar management because stress triggers the release of cortisol and adrenaline into the bloodstream and these hormones increase blood sugar. We also know that beyond the physiological effects of stress – like inflammation, skin problems and decreased gut health – chronic stress can lead to depression. Have too much of this kind of scenario and your health is definitely going to be compromised. However, while the classic Australian methods of de-stressing like eating, drinking and collapsing in front of the TV are popularly thought to offer stress relief, they often just make things worse. Simply because when we're stressed, we often make poor choices as to how and what we do to feel better.

> *'Tension is who you think you should be. Relaxation is who you are.'*
> **Chinese proverb**

Relaxation can be defined as the state of being free from mental stress and muscular tension through either conscious effort or a process that decreases the wear and tear of everyday life challenges on your mind and body. So, let's start this challenge with an experiment... YOU!

Welcome to my Islands of Bliss™ Relaxation Challenge!

All you have to do is set aside 20 minutes a day for a month to consciously take time out to relax. At the end of one month shoot me an email to *suzanna@islandsofbliss.com* and tell me how things have changed for you. By the way, my business name – **'Islands of Bliss'** – is no accident. Its entire purpose is to remind people to take some pleasurably relaxing time out.

15 Ways You Can Start Relaxing Today

The following are some ways to relax and why they work. Pick one or several. Try a different one every day for the whole month if you like. The rules are simple: no phone calls, social media or internet browsing while you're relaxing.

(1) Breathe out: Take a step back when you feel yourself getting upset or anxious. Step back psychologically and physically, if possible. Then observe your breathing. If you're breathing rapidly or barely breathing at all, these are the signs of stress. Relax by breathing slowly out and then slowly in.

THE BODY CONNECTION

(2) Laugh: Watch or read a comedy. Share a joke. Laughter is very good for you. A good laugh lowers blood pressure, reduces stress hormones, improves cardiac health, boosts your immune system, triggers the release of feel-good hormones called endorphins, relaxes the whole body and produces a general sense of wellbeing.

(3) Spend time with your dog or cat: It's well known that spending time with a pet can improve wellbeing and reduce feelings of stress. Dogs are the ultimate forgiveness teachers. Cats are wonderful meditation teachers. Even rabbits, guinea pigs, mice and budgies help alleviate anxiety and stress. And getting together with other pet owners for a lively chat about your pet's eccentricities and behaviour is a wonderful salve for the stress of loneliness.

(4) Listen to soothing music: Research shows that listening to music can reduce anxiety, depression, blood pressure and pain. Listening to music also improves sleep quality, mood, memory, improves learning and concentration and even helps delay brain ageing.

(5) Spend time in nature: A recent study on the 'urban nature experience' found that taking as little as 20 minutes out of your day to stroll or sit in a place that makes you feel in contact with nature can significantly lower stress hormone levels. If you're lucky enough to live in the country take advantage of it. If you're a city dweller, seek out a tree or a place where the birds sing. Nature is all around you wherever you are.

(6) Soak in a warm bath: Not only does a warm bath soothe joint pain and sore muscles, it can also greatly improve your mood as you give yourself over to warmth and pleasure. The steam from a warm bath acts as a natural decongestant by encouraging you to breathe more deeply and slowly – which also lowers anxiety and irritation. A few drops of calming essential oils such a lavender, sandalwood, chamomile or rose can elevate the experience to sublime.

(7) Go for a walk: Walking boosts your mood and helps relieve depression and anxiety because it leads your body to produce and release endorphins – which act as natural painkillers, improve your ability to sleep and reduce stress. Walking can also make a very real difference to your ability to cope with anxiety.

(8) Go for a swim: Science has long known there are measurable benefits to being in or near water. There's growing interest in the idea that swimming can reduce stress more so than other sports. Like all forms of exercise, swimming releases endorphins in your brain, increasing positivity and bringing about a sense of wellbeing.

(9) Go for a massage: There is nothing quite like a classic aromatherapy massage with soothing essential oils to de-stress your body, mind and spirit. Massage lowers blood pressure while increasing circulation; it makes you aware of your body in the most pleasurable and relaxing way.

(10) Do yoga or Tai Chi: People who practice Tai Chi and yoga experience less anxiety and stress. You could say that both yoga and Tai Chi are perfect blends of challenge and relaxation. Both disciplines improve breath control, awareness, meditation focus and cognitive functions. Confidence and wellbeing are also enhanced with the improvement of coordination, balance, flexibility and strength.

(11) Bake a loaf of bread: An unusual addition to a list of relaxation modalities but I've never met a person who made their own bread who *wasn't* relaxed! At least while making it. Forget about the automatic bread-maker machine! All that mixing and kneading can be wonderfully soothing. The smell of freshly baking bread is known to relax people. And there's something very satisfying about slicing into a freshly baked loaf you've made with your own hands.

(12) Learn how to meditate: Meditation is a habitual process of training your mind to focus and redirect your thoughts. It helps you get off the mouse-wheel of stress and anxiety caused by 'overthinking'. You can learn meditation in a class or through a podcast. You can also try guided meditation where you relax to a CD or MP3 designed to guide you through the process step by step. *(See my special reader* *offers for the 'Islands of Bliss' Relaxation and Sleep Guided Meditations at the end of this book.)*

(13) Grow something: Creating a herb or vegetable garden can be both rewarding and relaxing. Once established, maintenance can be your daily meditation as you watch your seedlings grow into useful and tasty foods and flavourings. Growing and tending plants, whether in a garden, courtyard or balcony brings you into contact with the rhythms of nature which are well known to be relaxing.

(14) Don't sweat the small stuff: Some people get stressed sitting in bumper-to-bumper traffic, worrying about being late or not being able to do what they'd planned in the time they'd allowed. Others simply take the time to sit back, listen to music and appreciate the break as much needed quiet time. That too can be your 20 minutes of peace, if you let it.

(15) Give up being perfect: Let's face it, when you pressure yourself to achieve perfection, you set yourself up for failure. Especially in certain areas of life like housework, cooking, comparing how your life is stacking up against your peers and whether or not you're *'red carpet Insta-ready'*. When you stress about failure or under-achievement, you find yourself worrying at every step that you'll make a mistake. But making mistakes is far better than faking perfection, anyway. Many wonderful inventions and achievements have occurred simply because a mistake illuminated some vital element which wouldn't have been noticed otherwise. The trick is to strive for progress rather than perfection. And that goes for your relaxation routine too.

> *'One of the basic rules of the universe is that nothing is perfect. Perfection simply doesn't exist... Without imperfection neither you nor I would exist.'*
>
> **Stephen Hawking**

CHAPTER 12

And So, To Sleep...

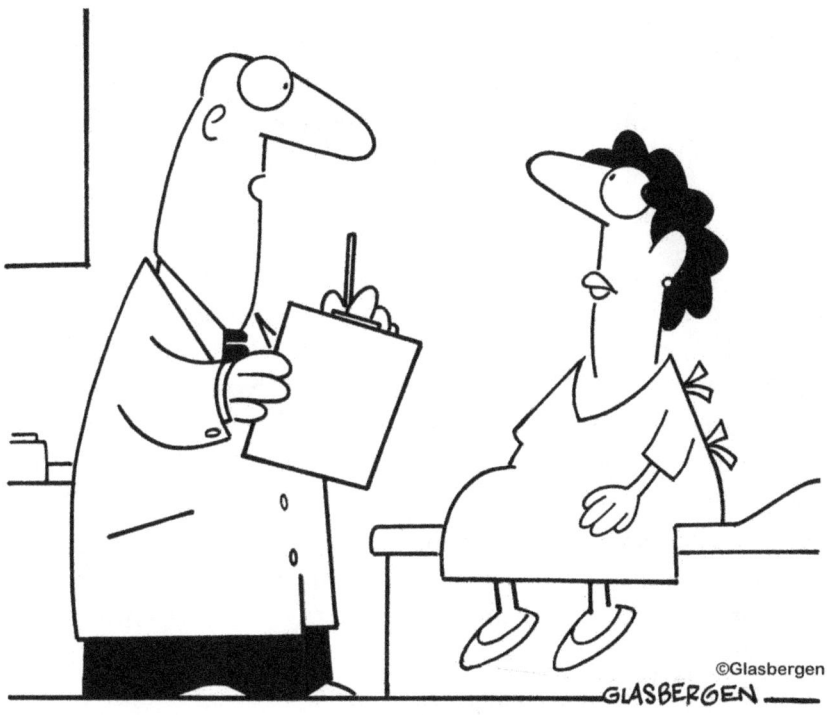

"If you have trouble falling asleep, lick your feet for a few minutes. It works for my cat!"

We live in sleepless times, folks. Rampant disruption, warp speed change on almost every level of our business, private and social lives. A 24-hour news churn and commentary which often confuses bloviation with information. So-called 'connectivity efficiencies' that keep us plugged in 24/7. Workers expected to behave and perform like machines lest they be replaced by robots or contractors willing to perform like them. Stratospheric executive bonuses funded by downsizing, tax-dodging, price-gouging and mega-mergers – while the rest of us get to grips with the gig economy and doing more with less as inflation outstrips frozen wages. No wonder burnout, anxiety and depression are on the rise. And hardly surprising Australia has an officially declared sleep problem. Because all the above represents more profound change in little more than 20 years than we've seen in the past 100 and many are struggling to keep up. For what it's worth we're not alone either. The entire Western world is in the grip of the biggest insomnia epidemic since the London Blitz because so many of us still haven't got the hang of sleeping with one eye open.

The one certainty we can definitely rely on though, is that if there's money to be made, there are a lot of people who couldn't give a rat's razoo about the trail of destruction increasingly left by socially thoughtless, selfish practices employed to achieve that one single goal. The battle to the top fuelled by allowing the environment and fellow human beings to fall to the bottom with often calamitous consequences. So, could it be that another reason Australians are battling insomnia and its unhealthy outfall is that, in our heart of hearts, we all know that the relentlessly self-interested, man-made pressures we've adopted as 'the new normal' are simply not sustainable? Especially when these pressures are increasing exponentially in direct proportion to expectations of corporate quarterlies and annual profits which are also expected to increase forever and ever, amen.

> *'Just like obesity, smoking, drinking too much and not exercising enough, sleep problems cause real harm in our community. It's high time we moved this issue off the backburner to the forefront of national thinking.*
>
> *There is a false belief shared by a lot of us that sleep is a waste of time and that we can get away with less than we really need, but the truth is people who cut corners with their sleep function below their best. They are not as mentally sharp, as vigilant, as attentive or as patient as they would otherwise be.'*
>
> **Dr. David Hillman,
> director of the Sleep Health Foundation**

We've already talked about the dodgy consumer practices of Big Food in this book. But what about the dodgy consumer practices of Big Tech? There's much in the news these days about how the algorithm business is out of control. Apps that track our every move. Privacy down the drain. Computer games designed to be every bit as addictive as fast food. Way back in 1994, who knew that one of the biggest disruptors across every facet of our lives would be our then dinky little mobile phones? Who even remembers that Facebook is only 15 years old? That Google is only 20 years old? Who could have predicted that many of us would be taking our phones to bed with us – for shopping, hooking up, scrolling and emailing? And what on earth possessed Apple in 2019 to promote 'The longest battery life in an iPhone ever' by showing people conking out in their beds and offices while their iPhone X carries on without them? But here we are, overstimulated by blue light, using sleep pattern apps to measure how long it takes us to fall asleep and whether we're staying there (or not) instead of… well, just flopping into our cots, maybe having a little read of a real book with real pages or even (gasp!) sex with our overtired partners before… *tah dah!*... falling asleep naturally.

> *'Overall, 44 per cent of adults are on the internet just before bed almost every night and 59 per cent of these late-night workers, web surfers, movie watchers or online gamers have more than two sleep problems. The result is a less productive, less safe and less pleasant work and family environment… Accident risk goes up, workplace performance goes down and your mood, your heart and your blood pressure can all be affected.'*
> **Dr. David Hillman,
> director of the Sleep Health Foundation**

There is no mystery as to why sleep deprivation has long been one of the most effective forms of torture, worldwide. However – although sleep deprivation is certainly effective in breaking the spirit, confusing the mind, destroying physical health, obliterating accurate memory, eliminating coherent speech and eventually causing hallucinations – it's well known that this particular method of torture isn't conducive to extracting useful information out of anyone. Simply because the likelihood of gaining 'actionable intelligence' diminishes the longer a subject is deprived of sleep.

> 'A mind tortured to that extremity will not provide anything that can be trusted as relevant to the real world. Even if the person really knew some vital bit of information (e.g. the location of a ticking time bomb), prolonged sleep deprivation will make it less likely the person could accurately and meaningfully communicate that information. Beyond a certain point the sleep deprived individual can no longer maintain enough cognitive coherence to say anything useful to anyone.'
> **Kelly Bulkeley,**
> **'Why Sleep Deprivation is Torture',**
> *Psychology Today,* **December 15, 2014**

And then, way back in the 16th century 'witch-hunts' of Scotland:

> '... civilians participated in several nationwide witch-hunts. At the height of sorcery and witch hysteria, women who allegedly practised witchcraft were captured and trialled. The civilians needed a confession from the accused before a conviction, and thus "waking the witch" was born. It involved depriving the woman of sleep for days, after which they would begin to hallucinate. The things captured women said and did during these hallucinations were interpreted as their "confessions" – today, we might describe such incidents as psychotic episodes – and as such the women were convicted of witchcraft. Sounds somewhat preposterous, doesn't it? But in those days, mass hysteria – the phenomenon that transmits the "illusion of threat" through society – was fuelled by fear, rumours, and panic.'
> **From 'Sleep deprivation… as a form of torture',**
> *Optalert* **website, January 24th, 2017**

Not only is sleep a basic biological necessity for humans, it's vital for all creatures on the planet. In short – we all need respite from the world to rest and repair by doing some serious sleeping, no matter what species we are.

So, you've got to marvel at sleep competitiveness, haven't you? Corporate high-flyers insisting they *never* get jetlag. Type-A business boffins who brag about sleeping a scant three hours a night in whatever time zone or conditions they find themselves. Management bigwigs wittering on about the worrying global productivity time-waste caused by lesser humans having to sleep at all. Self-proclaimed fatigue-free zones who set the company tone for the mass burnout of their employees. Right up there with the New Age virtue signalling from those who assume their good health, wealth and cancer-free lives are the sole result of their own spectacular worthiness.

> *'We have known the importance of sleep for decades yet for many reasons, sleep health has not received the attention it deserves within our community and in the health programs run by state and federal governments. In part this is because there are still many who think that it's a sign of "toughness" and a badge of honour to be able to get by on less sleep. The reality is that such an approach does harm – in some cases with very serious consequences.'*
>
> **Trent Zimmerman, MP, Chair's Foreword, 'Bedtime Reading', Inquiry into Sleep Health Awareness in Australia, House of Representatives Standing Committee on Health, Aged Care and Sport, April 2019, Canberra**

Maybe it's the chronic lack of sleep messin' with peoples' minds but when a phrase like *'I'll sleep when I'm dead'* gets defined in the online Urban Dictionary as *'having so much to do that sleep can only be accomplished in death'* – we should all be alarmed. *Very* alarmed. Especially given that:

- 90% of people with insomnia also have other negative health conditions

- Sleep disorders are often the precursor to heart disease, heart failure, irregular heartbeat, stroke, hypertension, obesity, diabetes, anxiety and depression

- Lack of sleep ages your skin and inhibits body repair, making you look and feel older than you are

- Poor sleep quality increases your chances of accidents, conflicts and poor decision making by at least 70%

- All your body's systems are negatively affected by the hormonal and repair imbalances of prolonged sleep deprivation.

Needless to say, late night yapping on your mobile, sleep competitiveness and the torturous stress of a world gone mad are not the only reasons why you can't get to sleep. Ask any new parent or shift-worker how they're doing at the beginning of whichever hour constitutes the start of their day. Bleary-eyed, exhausted and often memory-challenged, they're doing it tough, for sure. But while there's very little they can do about the incessant interruptions to their circadian rhythms, they are at least aware that they need to schedule in some shut-eye so they can function. So they can get at least one or two cycles of sleep per day. Because we don't just lie down and sleep. Like most things in life, even sleep is a process…

There are five different stages of sleep and we spend varying amounts of time in each one of them. Each sleep cycle takes around 110 minutes and then the cycle repeats itself.

Stage 1: The winding down stage. Also known as the transitional stage, in which it's easy to drift in and out of consciousness. During this non-rapid eye movement (non-REM) stage you may be partially awake while your mind begins to drift off. This period of drowsiness slowly leads to light sleep. Sometimes your muscles jerk, followed by a falling sensation which may jolt you back to consciousness.

Stage 2: The longest phase. Almost 50% of the time you spend asleep is in this stage. Stage two is also a non-REM phase and is one of the lighter stages of sleep. In stage two your heart rate slows and your core body temperature decreases. Your eye movements stop, and your brainwaves slow with the occasional burst of waves called 'sleep spindles'.

Stages 3 & 4: The deepest stages of sleep. These are the most difficult to wake up from. If you're rudely awakened from stages three and four, you'll be groggy and disoriented for several minutes (or even longer). These two stages are grouped together because they are periods of non-REM, slow wave sleep (SWS) – so called because your brain waves slow to delta waves with an occasional faster wave. As you move from stage three to stage four, the number of delta waves increase, and the faster waves decrease. Your blood pressure drops even further, your breathing becomes deeper and slower, your body becomes still. These are the most rejuvenating stages of sleep for your body. Hormones which aid growth, muscle and tissue repair and appetite control are released. In addition to the release of critical hormones, the blood flow to your muscles increases, bringing restorative oxygen and nutrients. It's also worth noting that stages three and four are also the stages when children (and sometimes adults) may experience nightmares, bedwetting and sleepwalking.

Stage 5: The only stage of rapid eye movement (REM). Rapid eye movement is so called because your eyes dart in various directions while your muscles are temporarily immobilised. Your breathing becomes shallow and irregular and your heart rate and blood pressure rise from previous levels. Also, unlike any of the other sleep stages, your brain is bursting with activity. We do most of our dreaming in stage five. During non-REM sleep, your mind rests while your body repairs. But in REM sleep your mind energises itself while your body is immobile. Neat, huh? While babies spend around 50% of their sleep time in REM, most adults spend about 20% of sleep in REM.

Although it's taken a little over 30 years to enter what may well come to be known as the 'Sleepless Age', disruption has always been with us and change has always been inevitable. And considering the speed at which they're both happening these days, we're just going to have to learn how to deal with them. Learn how to take care of ourselves when all our time-saving gadgets and upward mobility (or lack of it) are stripping away our rest and repair time. So, whatever the reasons or circumstances leading to your particular battle with sleep deprivation, here are some commonsense, natural ways to increase your chance of a good night's sleep and start making sleep a top priority in your health care regimen.

> 'Sleep is that golden chain that ties health and our bodies together.'
>
> **Thomas Dekker, writer (1572 – 1632)**

12 Things You *Can* Do to Help Yourself Get A Good Night's Sleep

(1) **Create firm boundaries around your sleep requirements.** Understand that sleep is not a waste of time. You've worked for it and you deserve it. Allow yourself the downtime of glorious sleep to repair your body, mind and spirit. Schedule what you need. After all, if you don't, who will?

(2) **Try to go to bed and get up around the same time each day.** Your body's circadian rhythm naturally aligns itself with sunrise and sunset. Studies have shown that irregular sleep habits can alter your circadian rhythm, as well as affecting your levels of melatonin, a key sleep hormone that tells your brain when it's time to relax and head for bed. Even going to bed late on the weekends can negatively affect those who already have insomnia.

(3) **Take a magnesium supplement an hour before bedtime.** Insomnia is a common symptom of magnesium deficiency. People with low magnesium often experience restless sleep and wake frequently during the night. Research indicates that supplemental magnesium can improve relaxation and enhance sleep quality. Magnesium glycinate is one of the most absorbable forms of magnesium and is known to raise overall levels fairly quickly. Follow the instructions on the packaging and take your dose an hour or two before bedtime.

(4) **Ask your doctor about a melatonin supplement.** In one study, 2mg of melatonin before bed helped people fall asleep faster, and improved sleep quality and energy the next day. Melatonin can also be useful when travelling and adjusting to new time zones as it helps your body's circadian rhythm to reset and return to normal.

(5) **Eat a starchy dinner or late snack.** In one study a high-carb meal eaten four hours before bed helped people fall asleep faster. Although I can personally confirm the small starchy snack strategy, interestingly, another study found that a low-carb dietary regimen also improved sleep. Obviously, a 'snack' is different from a 'dietary regimen' though. So, if you need a quick remedy, try a cracker or half a banana. Some people swear by hot milk with honey. Experiment to see what works best for you.

(6) **Relax and clear your mind in the evening.** While I understand that not everyone can start winding down precisely at sunset, setting boundaries around at least the hour before you go to sleep is important.

(7) **Banish screens from your bedroom.** Make love, read a book, listen to music, count backwards from 100… anything that doesn't emit blue light or stress you out is better for your sleep habits than computer games, scrolling through social media or, god forbid, reading the news online.

(8) **Meditation and guided sleep preparation recordings.** The use of relaxation techniques before bed has been shown to improve sleep quality. They are also commonly used to treat insomnia. Listening to recordings (or music that helps you unwind) is a wonderfully soothing way to let go of your stresses and cares. *(See the special offers for my 'Islands of Bliss' relaxation and sleep recordings at the end of this book.)*

(9) **Increase bright light exposure during the day.** According to research, exposure to sunlight or bright artificial light during the daytime can improve the quality and duration of your sleep.

(10) **Stop watching TV and turn off bright lights at least an hour before bedtime.** Binge TV! We've all done it. Suddenly it's 1am and you're tossing up whether to watch just one more episode never mind that you can hardly keep your eyes open. It may seem harmless to veg in front of the TV – turn on, tune in, veg out – you and as many as two thirds of the world's adults with working TVs know that drill backwards. However, the combination of blue light with violence, gore and suspense will not help you sleep. And falling asleep on the couch doesn't count as a good night's sleep in anyone's book.

(11) **Take a warm lavender bath.** A relaxing warm bath an hour before bedtime can be just the thing you need to send you off to the land of nod. Whether you infuse fresh lavender flowers in a muslin bag or use a few drops of lavender essential oil, lavender is known to be soothing and calming addition to your pre-bedtime bath. Make sure you swish the essential oil around in the water to thoroughly disperse it before you step in. Then lie back and luxuriate... but not so much that you fall asleep in the bath. On second thoughts, maybe set an alarm.

(12) **When all else fails, invest in a few sessions of Cognitive Behavioural Therapy with a specialist sleep psychologist to help reset your sleep behaviour.** Research shows that CBT with a trained sleep psychologist can reduce chronic insomnia in around 70% of cases by prompting changes to sleep (and *pre*-sleep) behaviour and challenging negative thoughts.

12 Things That Definitely Won't Help You Get A Good Night's Sleep

(1) **An underlying sleep disorder.** If you've always struggled with poor sleep, it's wise to talk it over with your doctor. One common issue is sleep apnoea which causes interrupted, inconsistent breathing. People with this disorder stop breathing repeatedly while asleep. It's estimated that around 25% of men and 9% of women suffer from sleep apnoea, many of them undiagnosed.

(2) **Vigorous exercise before bedtime.** Although regular moderate to vigorous exercise is one of the best ways to improve your sleep and overall health, going hard just before sleep or even just late in the day can spoil your rest big-time. This is due to the stimulating effects of exercise which increase alertness and the hormones epinephrine and adrenaline. Try Tai Chi or yoga in the hours before bed if you want exercise that promotes relaxation and sleep.

(3) **Spicy, heavy, sugary or XXL meals.** Late-night eating or large rich meals are known to negatively affect both sleep quality and melatonin production. Late night over-eating can also send you to bed with heartburn, indigestion and elevated body temperature. Too much candy, cake, chocolate or other sweet treats will also have you tossing and turning in bed as your body tries to work out what to do with all that sugar energy.

(4) **Smoking, vaping and nicotine substitutes.** Nicotine is a stimulant. It increases your heart rate and alertness, making you feel more awake when you least want to be. So, puffing or vaping away right up until bedtime is definitely not much use in the peaceful sleep stakes. Goes without saying that smoking cigarettes, cigars or a pipe in bed is both bad for you and a potential fire hazard.

(5) **Drinking large amounts of liquid before bed.** Shift workers, pilots, nurses, teachers, health workers and many other professionals often become dehydrated because they can't drink enough fluids during their day. If you find yourself desperately trying to quench your thirst at the end of your day, you need to reassess your hydration habits. Trying to fit it all in before bedtime can have you up all night running to the loo.

(6) **Caffeine.** A single shot of caffeine can stimulate your nervous system and enhance focus, energy and sports performance. A double shot espresso can either rev you up for the day or send you into an anxiety tailspin, complete with palpitations. So, it's obvious why you should avoid caffeine in all forms at bedtime or pretty much any time after 4pm at the latest. Individuals vary, though. One study showed that consuming caffeine within six hours of bedtime significantly worsened sleep quality. Another showed caffeine merely shortened overall sleep time. Yet another showed caffeine prevented the smooth transition to sleep. The sensible upshot? If you do crave the taste of coffee as a pick-me-up late in the day, stick with the decaffeinated variety and avoid all three roads to sleeplessness.

(7) **Blue light.** No, not the garden fairy lights. Electronic devices like smartphones and computers emit blue light in large amounts. Blue light tricks your body into thinking it's daytime. Apps that block blue light are available for both iPhones and Android models. Apps such as *f.lux* will block blue light on your laptop or computer.

(8) **Catching up on your emails in bed.** This activity comes under the heading of setting clear boundaries around your own needs. Some countries even have rules around the hours employees can be expected to receive and answer business emails.

AND SO, TO SLEEP...

(9) **Alcohol.** No matter how warm and sleepy you may feel after a couple stiff ones after dinner, booze-induced sleep is not quality shut-eye. Alcohol is known to both cause and increase the symptoms of sleep apnoea and snoring. Late-night alcohol consumption also reduces night-time melatonin production and leads to disrupted sleep patterns. Reducing or eliminating alcohol consumption in the evenings particularly benefits those who are regularly woken up around 4am as their livers start work on processing the sugars of their nightly tipples.

(10) **An uncomfortable bed.** Have you ever wondered why you sleep better in a hotel? Making sure people get a good night's sleep is their core business. The better quality of their bedding, the more soundly people sleep, the better their reviews. Maybe it's time for *you* to learn from the professionals and invest in a new mattress and new pillows. Especially if you're tossing about all night or waking up with back, shoulder and neck pain. You'll certainly achieve a better quality of sleep when you review and upgrade your bedding like a pro.

(11) **Long daytime naps.** While short power naps can be beneficial (especially for new parents!), anything over 30 minutes can interfere with your night-time sleep. Long daytime naps can also leave you feeling groggy, disoriented and cranky – a condition known as 'sleep inertia'. Needless to say, it's an individual process. You may need to adopt a trial and error approach while you work out the nap time that's good for you, especially if you need to be fully alert when you wake up.

(12) **A noisy, messy bedroom with glowing electronic devices etc.** Optimise your sleeping space by transforming it into a clean, comfortable and peaceful pod that encourages deep relaxation. Get rid of the clutter. Block external lights and noise. Reduce or eliminate artificial light from gadgets

and alarm clocks. Do whatever you can to regulate the temperature to around 20C (or whatever temperature feels right for you).

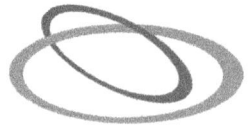

"No more words.

In the name of this place we drink in with our breathing, stay quiet like a flower.

So the nightbirds will start singing."

~ Rumi ~

AFTERWORD

Wellbeing is a journey, not an app...

Congratulations on making the decision to read this book and improve your health and wellbeing. I hope that along the way you've picked up some new ideas and reconnected with your own marvellous common sense. I also hope I've helped you expand your knowledge and eliminated some of the fictions around the subject of taking better care of yourself in a world that seems to be spinning faster and faster.

It's been an absolute pleasure to share some of my self-care knowledge with you. So, while you still have this book open... how about considering improving your health and lifestyle choices one chapter at a time? What if you took each chapter and turned it into a mini course for your chosen health update for a week? Or a month? By the end of 12 weeks... or 12 months... your entire self-care routine could be completely revamped! *In fact, if you covered two chapters a week, you could be transformed in just six weeks!*

You could be feeling so much better – with more energy and the kind of aliveness that comes with being in control of your own healthy habits, never mind what's happening at home or at work. The most important thing is that you take *action*, no matter how small at first. Follow through on your commitment to yourself. Recommit when things go haywire. And always remember that the best things in life – *resolve, kindness, faith, resilience, strength, a sense of humour, fortitude, determination, courage, curiosity, effort and grit* – are not only free... they're *analog*!

Further reading

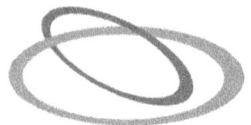

- *Come Of Age: The Case for Elderhood in a Time of Trouble*
  - Stephen Jenkinson (North Atlantic, 2018)

- *Irresistible: The Rise of Addictive Technology and the Business of Keeping Us Hooked* - Adam Alter (Penguin Press, 2017)

- *Affluenza: When Too Much Is Never Enough*
  - Clive Hamilton & Richard Denniss (Allen & Unwin, 2005)

- *Gut: The Inside Story of Our Body's Most Underrated Organ*
  - Giulia Enders (Scribe, 2015)

- *Natural Causes: Life, Death and the Illusion of Control*
  - Barbara Ehrenreich (Granta, 2018)

- *Sapiens. A Brief History of Humankind*
  - Yuval Noah Harari (Harper, 2015)

- *Why Mindfulness is Better than Chocolate*
  - David Michie (Allen & Unwin, 2014)

FURTHER READING

- *Being Mortal: Medicine and What Matters in the End*
  - Atul Gawande (Profile Trade, 2015)

- *Grit: Why Passion and Resilience are the Secrets to Success*
  - Angela Duckworth (Vermilion, 2017)

- **The Trauma of Everyday Life**
  - Mark Epstein, MD (Penguin Books, 2014)

- *How to Live Like Your Cat*
  - Stéphane Garnier (Harper Collins, 2017)

- *5 Ingredients: Quick & Easy Food*
  - Jamie Oliver (Michael Joseph, 2017)

- *Vegan in 7: Delicious Plant-Based Recipes in 7 Ingredients or Fewer* - Rita Serano (Kyle Books, 2018)

- *Shit You Don't Need*
  - Dillie Keane (https://shityoudontneed.blog)

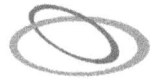

About the Author

Suzanna Hammond was born in Melbourne to actor parents. She spent her early years in Europe and England, returning to Australia to attend her seventh school as a 'ten-pound Pom'.

By the age of five she was already interested in healing. Her first patients were half-frozen hedgehogs, sparrows and water birds plucked from English winter snow and other hazards. Thus, began her lifelong interest in the often astonishing results of the ancient method of 'laying on of hands'.

Following a writing career in media and advertising – ended by a life-changing medical rescue and subsequent 'life path' epiphany – she began formal training in aromatherapy and other massage therapies, as well as somatics, bioenergetics, Feldenkrais techniques and natural skincare. To finance her career change she spent several years writing pharmaceutical advertising and 10 years writing and producing perinatal education videos for new mothers and maternity hospitals. Later, she added reiki, lifestyle coaching and fitness training to the mix. She has been a student of Tai Chi and various schools of yoga for many years.

Suzanna is well known in Sydney's Inner West as a holistic healer and 'People Renovator'. Her studio business, **Islands of Bliss**, specialises in training and treatment across a variety of mind/body modalities including transformational and remedial bodywork, aromatherapy, remedial skin care, pain relief nutrition, stress management, Tai Chi falls prevention and strength training for the over 50s. She also practices reiki across a variety of species, including cats, dogs, horses, birds, lizards, possums, fish and humans.

Suzanna currently lives in a 100-year-old tram driver's cottage set in a lush garden designed as a wildlife corridor in the middle of suburbia. Her many passions include her clients, her 'flock' of Lhasa Apsos (Tibetan lamasery dogs) and the communicative art of simplifying complex information.

Acknowledgements

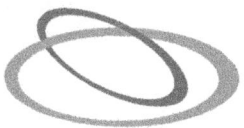

To my clients – past and present – thank you for inviting me into your lives and entrusting me with your injuries, recoveries, maintenance, hopes and dreams. I have learned more from you than you will ever know, and I am a better therapist for the experience.

My heartfelt appreciation to my beautiful and generous band of forward readers – Annette Livesey, E. Joy Bowles PhD, Juliette Knight and Vonnie Selhofer. Your knowledge, humour, encouragement, attention to detail, criticism, forbearance and fearlessness have been invaluable in the writing of this book.

Special thanks to my adventurous and committed publishers – Natasa and Stuart Denman @ Ultimate World Publishing. Many thanks to the wonderful all-round 'den-mother', Vivienne Mason; my front cover designer, Nikola Boskovski; and my copyeditor Marinda Wilkinson.

SUZANNA HAMMOND - YOUR NEXT EVENT SPEAKER

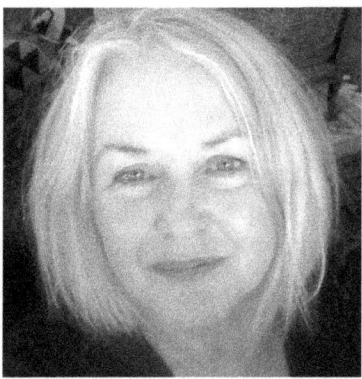

With over 30 years of experience as a wellness & bodywork practitioner, Suzanna brings an informative, practical and lighthearted touch to upgrading mental and physical self-care in the digital age.

An engaging and passionate speaker, Suzanna delivers her content with humour, charm and wit – captivating her audiences with her simple, yet life-changing presentations.

Suzanna is available to speak to groups, seminars, workshops & wellness industry trainings on:

- Analog strategies for burnout , busy-ness & borborygmi
- Exploding the Magic Silver Bullet
- The food lover's guide to pain relief
- Saving face – the beauty spa in your kitchen
- Forget about the house – let's renovate YOU!

Contact Suzanna at suzanna@islandsofbliss.com to discuss subjects, availability and rates.

Depending on location & availability, Suzanna may speak at non-profit events free of charge.

Special offer for readers of

'THE BODY CONNECTION
an Analog ReBoot for Digital Times'

2 SOOTHING MEDITATIONS for REST & SLEEP

* MP3 downloads AUS$15   Save $10!

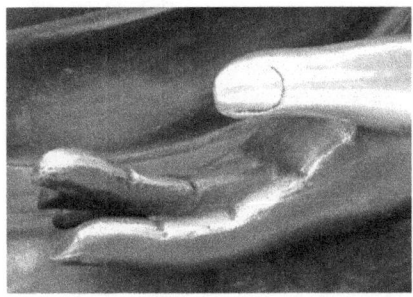

What people are saying:

'The most relaxing way to dial down, kick back & chill out I've found...'

'The perfect lunch time relaxation reboot for busy people...'

'No way you can't sleep at night after 10 minutes of this... brilliant!'

Go to –

www.islandsofbliss.com.au

FREE GIFT!

FOR READERS OF

'THE BODY CONNECTION
an Analog ReBoot for Digital Times'

'21 FOODS A DAY'

3 delicious days of recipes
Start improving your nutrition today!

Visit –

www.islandsofbliss.com.au

FOR YOUR **FREE** DOWNLOAD

DISCLAIMER

All of the information, concepts and advice contained within this publication are of general comment only and are not in any way intended as individual advice. The intent is to offer a variety of information to provide a wider range of choices now and in the future, recognising that we all have widely diverse skills, abilities, circumstances and viewpoints. While all attempts have been made to verify information provided in this publication, neither the author nor the publisher nor the marketing agents assumes any responsibility for errors, omissions or contrary interpretation of the subject matter whatsoever under any condition or circumstances. Should any reader choose to make use of the information contained herein, this is their decision. It is recommended that the reader obtain their own independent advice and where medical matters are involved, they should firstly consult with their relevant medical practitioner prior to embarking on any information contained within this book.

Where client stories have been used, names and circumstances have been changed to protect privacy.

www.ingramcontent.com/pod-product-compliance
Lightning Source LLC
Chambersburg PA
CBHW031152020426
42333CB00013B/635